Children's Interview for Psychiatric Syndromes

Scoring Forms

PARENT VERSION

AF753713

P-ChIPS

Also available from American Psychiatric Publishing Group (1-800-368-5777; www.appi.org)

- **ChIPS—Children's Interview for Psychiatric Syndromes** (Order #8398)
(reusable interview administration booklet)

Based on strict DSM-IV criteria and validated in more than 12 years of studies, the ChIPS is brief and simple to administer. Questions are succinct, simply worded, and easily understood by children and adolescents. Practitioners in clinical and research settings alike have already found the ChIPS indispensable in screening for conditions such as attention-deficit/hyperactivity disorder, conduct disorder, substance abuse, phobias, anxiety disorders, stress disorders, eating disorders, mood disorders, elimination disorders, and schizophrenia.

Scoring Form for ChIPS, package of 20 (Order #8846)
(one-time-use booklet for recording answers, with Profile Sheet)

Scoring Forms provide ample space for recording verbatim responses to interview questions, with check boxes to indicate whether symptom criteria and duration and impairment requirements are met. A Profile Sheet, perforated for easy removal from the Scoring Form, is included to itemize principal findings and diagnoses.

Report Form for ChIPS, package of 20 (Order #8899)
(one-time-use abbreviated summary form)

Report Forms provide a quick way of conveying ChIPS results. If subsequently desired, this "at-a-glance" summary of the symptoms endorsed during the interview can be used by a clinician to identify areas warranting further scrutiny.

- **P-ChIPS—Children's Interview for Psychiatric Syndromes—Parent Version** (Order #8847)
(reusable interview administration booklet)

The Parent Version of the ChIPS essentially consists of the same interview text altered from second to third person to address the parent rather than the child (e.g., "Have you ever" is changed to "Has your child ever").

Scoring Form for P-ChIPS, package of 20 (Order #8396)
(one-time-use booklet for recording answers, with Profile Sheet)

Report Form for P-ChIPS, package of 20 (Order #8399)
(one-time-use abbreviated summary form)

- **Administration Manual** (Order #8849)

Covering both the ChIPS and the P-ChIPS, the Administration Manual is informative and user-friendly. It presents background information about the interview's development, detailed instructions for conducting the interview and recording its results, explicit criteria for assessing interviewee responses, complete specifications for preparing mental health paraprofessionals to administer the interview, and illustrative case studies.

ISBN 978-0-88048-396-4

90000

9 780880 483964

AMERICAN PSYCHIATRIC ASSOCIATION PUBLISHING

P-ChIPS Scoring Form
Profile Sheet

Child's Number: ____________________ Date: ____________

Child's Name: ____________________ Time Started: ____________

Date of Birth: ____________ Age: ____________ Time Ended: ____________

Race: ____________ Sex: ____________ Interviewer: ____________

Informant's Name: ____________________

Informant's Relationship (circle one): Mother, Father, Stepmother, Stepfather, Guardian, Other: ____________

	Disorder	Symptoms	Diagnosis	Duration	Clinician's Diagnosis
ADHD	**Attention-Deficit/Hyperactivity Disorder**	<>	<>	<>	**Axis I**
	Type: Inattentive, Hyperactive–Impulsive, Combined				
ODD	**Oppositional Defiant Disorder**	<>	<>	<>	
CD	**Conduct Disorder**	<>	<>	<>	
	Onset: Childhood, Adolescent				
	Severity: Mild, Moderate, Severe				
SUBAB	**Substance Abuse**	<>	<>	<>	
	Substance(s): ____________				
PHO	**Specific Phobia**	<>	<>	<>	**Axis II**
	Type: ____________				
SOCPHO	**Social Phobia**	<>	<>	<>	
SEPANX	**Separation Anxiety Disorder**	<>	<>	<>	**Axis III**
GENANX	**General Anxiety Disorder**	<>	<>	<>	
OCD	**Obsessive-Compulsive Disorder**	<>	<>	<>	
PTSD	**Posttraumatic Stress Disorder**	<>	<>	<>	**Axis IV**
	Type: Acute, Chronic				
	Onset: Regular, Delayed				
ASD	**Acute Stress Disorder**	<>	<>	<>	
ANO	**Anorexia**	<>	<>	<>	**Axis V**
BUL	**Bulimia**	<>	<>	<>	**current:**
DEP	**Major Depressive Disorder**	<>	<>	<>	**past year:**
DYS	**Dysthymic Disorder**	<>	<>	<>	
MAN	**Mania**	<>	<>	<>	
HYPOMAN	**Hypomania**	<>	<>	<>	
ENU	**Enuresis**	<>	<>	<>	
	Type: Nocturnal, Diurnal, Both				
ENC	**Encopresis**	<>	<>	<>	
SCZ	**Schizophrenia**	<>	<>	<>	
PSY	**Psychosis**	<>	<>	<>	

Psychosocial Stressors:

Other Stressors:

Behavioral Observations

Appearance:

Affect:

Effort:

Level of Activity:

Unusual Behaviors:

Presenting Problem

Home

1.

2.

School

1.

2.

3.

4.

5.

Peers/Work

1.

2.

3.

4.

5.

Medication

Type:

Dosage:

Child's Name: ______________________________

Date: ______________

ADHD	ODD	CD
A. Inattention 1. <a> <b> 2. < > 3. <a> <b> 4. <a> <b> <c> 5. < > 6. < > 7. < > 8. <a> <b> 9. <a> <b> B. Hyperactivity–Impulsivity 1. <a> <b> 2. <a> <b> 3. < > 4. <a> <b> 5. < > 6. <a> <b> 7. < > 8. <a> <b> 9. <a> <b> <c>	1. <a> <b> 2. <a> <b> 3. <a> <b> <c> <d> 4. < > 5. <a> <b> 6. < > 7. < > 8. < >	1. < > 2. <a> <b> 3. < > 4. < > 5. < > 6. < > 7. <a> <b> 8. <a> <b> 9. < > 10. <a> <b> 11. < > 12. < > 13. < > 14. < > 15. <a> <b>
Criteria If ≥6 in *A only*, then criteria met Inattentive < > If ≥6 in *B only*, then criteria met Hyperactive–Impulsive < > If ≥6 in A *and* ≥6 in B, then criteria met Combined < >	**Criteria** If ≥4, then criteria met ODD < >	**Criteria** If ≥3, then criteria met CD < >
Duration 1. __________ (years old) 2. < > ________ (years old) 3. < > ________ (months) * DUR met for ADHD < >	**Duration** 1. __________ (years old) 2. < > ________ (years old) 3. < > ________ (months) * DUR met for ODD < >	**Duration** 1. __________ (years old) 2. < > ________ (years old) 3. < > ________ (months) * DUR met for CD < >
Impairment 1. < > home 2. < > school 3. < > peers	**Impairment** 1. < > home 2. < > school 3. < > peers	**Impairment** 1. < > home 2. < > school 3. < > peers **Type** Childhood Onset < > Adolescent Onset < > Mild < > Moderate < > Severe < >

SUB AB

1. < >
   <a>____________________
   <b>____________________
   <c>____________________
   ____
2. < > ____________________
3. < > ____________________
4. < > ____________________

Duration
1. __________ (years old)
2. < > __________ (years old)
   __________ (months)

* DUR met for SUB AB < >

Impairment
1. <a> <b>
2. < >
3. <a> <b>
4. < >

Criteria
If any use (Q1–4) and any impairment (1–4), then criteria met SUB AB < >

Type(s) ____________________
____
____
____

PHO

1. ____________________
   ____
   ____
2. <a> <b>
3. <a> <b>
4. <ai> <aii> <aiii> <aiv> <b>
5. <a> <b>

Criteria
If 1–4, then criteria met PHO < >

Duration
1. __________ (years old)
2. < > __________ (years old)
3. < > __________ (months)

* DUR met for PHO < >

Impairment
1. < > home
2. < > school
3. < > peers

Type(s)

Animal	< >
Natural Environment	< >
Blood–Injection–Injury	< >
Situational	< >
Other ________________	< >

SOCIAL PHO

1. <a> <b>
2. < >
3. <a> <b>
4. <ai> <aii> <aiii> <aiv> <b>
5. < >

Criteria
If 1–4, then criteria met SOCIAL PHO < >

Duration
1. __________ (years old)
2. < > __________ (years old)
3. < > __________ (months)

*DUR met for SOCIAL PHO < >

Impairment
1. < > home
2. < > school
3. < > peers

SEP ANX	GEN ANX	OCD
1. <a> <b> 2. <a> <b> 3. < > 4. <a> <b> 5. <a> <b> 6. <a> <b> 7. <a> <b> 8. <a> <b>	1. < > ______________ ______________ ______________ ______________ ______________ 2. <a> <b> 3. <a> <b> <c> <d> <e> <f>	A. Compulsions 1. < > ______________ 2. <a> ______________ <b> 3. < > B. Obsessions 1. <a> ______________ <b> ______________ <c> ______________ 2. <a> <b> <c> 3. < > C. Interference 1. <a> <b> <c>
Criteria If ≥3, then criteria met SEP ANX < >	**Criteria** If 1–3, then criteria met GEN ANX < >	**Criteria** If A1, A2, & C, then criteria met Compulsions < > If B1, B2, & C, then criteria met Obsessions < > If Compulsions + and/or Obsessions +, then criteria met OCD < >
Duration 1. ______________ (years old) 2. < > __________ (years old) 3. < > __________ (weeks) *DUR met for SEP ANX < >	**Duration** 1. ______________ (years old) 2. < > __________ (years old) 3. < > __________ (months) *DUR met for GEN ANX < >	**Duration** 1. ______________ (years old) 2. < > __________ (years old) __________ (months) *DUR met for OCD < >
Impairment 1. < > home 2. < > school 3. < > peers	**Impairment** 1. < > home 2. < > school 3. < > peers	**Impairment** 1. < > home 2. < > school 3. < > peers

STRESS (ASD/PTSD)	ANO	BUL
A. Exposure 1. <a> <b> ____________ 2. <a> <b> <c> <d> <e> 3. < > ____________ B. Dissociation 1. <a> <b> <c> <d> 2. < > 3. < > 4. < > 5. < > C. Reexperiencing 1. <a> <b> <c> 2. <a> <b> 3. <a> <b> 4. <a> <b> 5. < > D. Avoidance 1. <a> <b> 2. <a> <b> <c> 3. < > 4. <a> <b> 5. <a> <b> 6. <a> <b> 7. <a> <b> E. Hyperarousal 1. <a> <b> 2. <a> <b> 3. < > 4. < > 5. < >	1. <a> <b> 2. <a> ht: ____________ wt: ____________ <b> ht: ____________ wt: ____________ 3. <a> <b> <c> 4. <a> <b> <c> 5. < >	1. < > ____________ ____________ 2. <a> <b> <c> <d> 3. <a> <b> <c> <d> 4. <a> <b>
Criteria If A1 & A2, ≥3 in B, ≥1 in C, ≥3 in D, and ≥2 in E, then criteria met ASD < > If A1 & A2, ≥1 in C, ≥3 in D, and ≥2 in E, then criteria met PTSD < >	**Criteria** If 1–4 (&5 for pubescent girls), then criteria met ANO < >	**Criteria** If 1–4, then criteria met BUL < >
Duration 1. ____________ (years old) 2. < > ____________ (years old) 3. a. < > ________ (weeks) b. < > c. < > ________ (days) 4. < > ____________ (months) *DUR met for ASD < > *DUR met for PTSD < >	**Duration** 1. ____________ (years old) 2. < > ________ (years old) 3. < > ________ (months) *DUR met for ANO < >	**Duration** 1. ____________ (years old) 2. < > ________ (years old) 3. a. < > ______ (#/week) b. < > ______ (months) *DUR met for BUL < >
Impairment 1. < > home 2. < > school 3. < > peers **Type (PTSD)** Acute < > Regular Onset < > Chronic < > Delayed Onset < >	**Impairment** 1. < > home 2. < > school 3. < > peers	**Impairment** 1. < > home 2. < > school 3. < > peers

DEP/DYS (MDD/DD)

A. Dysphoric Mood
1. <a> <b> <c>
2. <a> <bi> <bii> <biii> <c> <d>

B. Loss of Interest
1. <a> <b>
2. <a> <b> <c>

C. Appetite Changes
1. <a> <b> <c>
2. <a> <b>

D. Sleep Changes
Bedtime: ________
Wakeup: ________
1. <a> <b> <c>
2. <a> <b>

E. Psychomotor Changes
1. <a> <b> <c> <d>
2. <a> <b>

F. Low Energy
1. <a> <b> <c> <d>

G. Guilt
1. <a> <b> <c> <d>
2. <a> <b>

H. Impaired Concentration
1. <a> <b> <c> <d> <e>
2. < >

I. Hopelessness
1. <a> <b> <c>

J. Morbid/Suicidal Thoughts
1. <a> <b>
2. <a> <b> <c> <d> <e>

____
____
____
____
____

DEP/DYS (MDD/DD)

Criteria

If A &/or B & ≥5 of A–H or J,
then criteria met
MDD < >

If A & ≥2 of C, D, F, G, H, or I,
then criteria met
DD < >

Duration

1. ____________ (years old)
2. < > ____________ (years old)
3. MDD < > ________ (weeks)
   DD < > ________ (months)

*DUR met for MDD < >
*DUR met for DD < >

Impairment

1. < > home
2. < > school
3. < > peers

MAN/HYPOMAN

A. Elevated Mood
1. <a> ____________
   <b> ____________
   <c> ____________
2. < > ____________

B. Other Symptoms
1. <a> ____________
   <b>
2. <a> <b> <c> ________
3. <a> <b> <c> <d>
4. <a> <b> <c>
5. < >
6. <a> <b> <c> <d> <e>
7. <a> <b> <c> <d>

C. Interference
1. < >
2. < >

Criteria

If A1(a, b, & c) + ≥3 in B + ≥1 in C
or
A2 + ≥4 in B + ≥1 in C,
then criteria met
MAN < >

If A1(a, b, & c) + ≥3 in B +
none in C
or
A2 + ≥4 in B + none in C,
then criteria met
HYPOMAN < >

Duration

1. ____________ (years old)
2. < > ____________ (years old)
3. MAN < > ________ (weeks)
   HYPO < > ________ (days)

*DUR met for MAN < >
*DUR met for HYPOMAN < >

Impairment

1. < > home
2. < > school
3. < > peers

ENU

1. < >
2. <a> <b>
3. <a> <b>

Criteria

If 1, ≥1 in 2, 3a, and 3b, then criteria met

ENU < >

Duration

1. ____________ (years old)
2. < > _________ (years old)
3. <a> _________ (x/week)
   <b> _________ (months)

*DUR met for ENU < >

Impairment

1. < > home
2. < > school
3. < > peers

Type

Nocturnal < >
Diurnal < >
Both < >

ENC

1. < >
2. < >

Criteria

If both 1 & 2, then criteria met

ENC < >

Duration

1. ____________ (years old)
2. < > _________ (years old)
3. <a> _________ (x/month)
   <b> _________ (months)

*DUR met for ENC < >

Impairment

1. < > home
2. < > school
3. < > peers

SCZ/PSY

A. Psychotic Symptoms
1. <a> <b> <c> <d> <e>
2. <a> <b> <c> <d> <e> <f>
3. < >
4. < >
5. < >

B. Interference
1. < >
2. < >
3. < >

Criteria

If ≥2 in A and ≥1 in B, then criteria met

SCZ < >

If ≥1 in A, then criteria met

PSY < >

Duration

1. ____________ (years old)
2. < > _________ (years old)
3. < > _________ (months)

*DUR met for SCZ < >
*DUR met for PSY < >

Impairment

1. < > home
2. < > school
3. < > peers

STRESSORS

A. Child Abuse/Neglect
1. <a> <b> <c>
2. <a> <b> <c> <d>
3. <a> <b> <c> <d>
4. < >
5. < >

Duration

1. ____________________
2. < > ____________________
3. ____________________
4. ____________________
5. < >

B. Other Stressors
1. <a> <b> <c> <d> <e>
2. < >
3. <a> <b>
4. <a> <b> <c>
5. <a> <b>
6. <a> <b>
7. <a> ________________
   <b>
8. <a> <b> <c> <d>
9. < > ________________
   ____
   ____
10. < >
11. < > ________________
   ____
   ____

P-ChIPS Scoring Form
Profile Sheet

Child's Number: ______________________________ Date: ______________

Child's Name: ______________________________ Time Started: ______________

Date of Birth: ______________ Age: ______________ Time Ended: ______________

Race: ______________ Sex: ______________ Interviewer: ______________

Informant's Name: ______________________________

Informant's Relationship (circle one): Mother, Father, Stepmother, Stepfather, Guardian, Other: ______________

	Disorder	Symptoms	Diagnosis	Duration	Clinician's Diagnosis
ADHD	**Attention-Deficit/Hyperactivity Disorder** *Type:* Inattentive, Hyperactive–Impulsive, Combined	<>	<>	<>	**Axis I**
ODD	**Oppositional Defiant Disorder**	<>	<>	<>	
CD	**Conduct Disorder** *Onset:* Childhood, Adolescent *Severity:* Mild, Moderate, Severe	<>	<>	<>	
SUBAB	**Substance Abuse** *Substance(s):* ______________	<>	<>	<>	
PHO	**Specific Phobia** *Type:* ______________	<>	<>	<>	**Axis II**
SOCPHO	**Social Phobia**	<>	<>	<>	
SEPANX	**Separation Anxiety Disorder**	<>	<>	<>	**Axis III**
GENANX	**General Anxiety Disorder**	<>	<>	<>	
OCD	**Obsessive-Compulsive Disorder**	<>	<>	<>	
PTSD	**Posttraumatic Stress Disorder** *Type:* Acute, Chronic *Onset:* Regular, Delayed	<>	<>	<>	**Axis IV**
ASD	**Acute Stress Disorder**	<>	<>	<>	
ANO	**Anorexia**	<>	<>	<>	**Axis V**
BUL	**Bulimia**	<>	<>	<>	**current:**
DEP	**Major Depressive Disorder**	<>	<>	<>	**past year:**
DYS	**Dysthymic Disorder**	<>	<>	<>	
MAN	**Mania**	<>	<>	<>	
HYPOMAN	**Hypomania**	<>	<>	<>	
ENU	**Enuresis** *Type:* Nocturnal, Diurnal, Both	<>	<>	<>	
ENC	**Encopresis**	<>	<>	<>	
SCZ	**Schizophrenia**	<>	<>	<>	
PSY	**Psychosis**	<>	<>	<>	

Psychosocial Stressors:

Other Stressors:

Behavioral Observations

Appearance:

Affect:

Effort:

Level of Activity:

Unusual Behaviors:

Presenting Problem

Home

1.

2.

School

1.

2.

3.

4.

5.

Peers/Work

1.

2.

3.

4.

5.

Medication

Type:

Dosage:

Child's Name: ______________________________

Date: ______________

ADHD	ODD	CD
A. Inattention 1. <a> <b> 2. < > 3. <a> <b> 4. <a> <b> <c> 5. < > 6. < > 7. < > 8. <a> <b> 9. <a> <b> B. Hyperactivity–Impulsivity 1. <a> <b> 2. <a> <b> 3. < > 4. <a> <b> 5. < > 6. <a> <b> 7. < > 8. <a> <b> 9. <a> <b> <c>	1. <a> <b> 2. <a> <b> 3. <a> <b> <c> <d> 4. < > 5. <a> <b> 6. < > 7. < > 8. < >	1. < > 2. <a> <b> 3. < > 4. < > 5. < > 6. < > 7. <a> <b> 8. <a> <b> 9. < > 10. <a> <b> 11. < > 12. < > 13. < > 14. < > 15. <a> <b>
Criteria If ≥6 in *A only*, then criteria met Inattentive < > If ≥6 in *B only*, then criteria met Hyperactive–Impulsive < > If ≥6 in A *and* ≥6 in B, then criteria met Combined < >	**Criteria** If ≥4, then criteria met ODD < >	**Criteria** If ≥3, then criteria met CD < >
Duration 1. ___________ (years old) 2. < > ________ (years old) 3. < > _________ (months) * DUR met for ADHD < >	**Duration** 1. ___________ (years old) 2. < > ________ (years old) 3. < > _________ (months) * DUR met for ODD < >	**Duration** 1. ___________ (years old) 2. < > ________ (years old) 3. < > _________ (months) * DUR met for CD < >
Impairment 1. < > home 2. < > school 3. < > peers	**Impairment** 1. < > home 2. < > school 3. < > peers	**Impairment** 1. < > home 2. < > school 3. < > peers **Type** Childhood Onset < > Adolescent Onset < > Mild < > Moderate < > Severe < >

SUB AB

1. < >
   <a>____________________
   <b>____________________
   <c>____________________
   ____
2. < > ____________________
3. < > ____________________
4. < > ____________________

Duration

1. ____________ (years old)
2. < > __________ (years old)
   __________ (months)

* DUR met for SUB AB < >

Impairment

1. <a> <b>
2. < >
3. <a> <b>
4. < >

Criteria

If any use (Q1–4) and any impairment (1–4), then criteria met SUB AB < >

Type(s) ____________________
____
____
____

PHO

1. ____________________
   ____
   ____
2. <a> <b>
3. <a> <b>
4. <ai> <aii> <aiii> <aiv> <b>
5. <a> <b>

Criteria

If 1–4, then criteria met PHO < >

Duration

1. ____________ (years old)
2. < > __________ (years old)
3. < > __________ (months)

* DUR met for PHO < >

Impairment

1. < > home
2. < > school
3. < > peers

Type(s)

Animal	< >
Natural Environment	< >
Blood–Injection–Injury	< >
Situational	< >
Other ________________	< >

SOCIAL PHO

1. <a> <b>
2. < >
3. <a> <b>
4. <ai> <aii> <aiii> <aiv> <b>
5. < >

Criteria

If 1–4, then criteria met SOCIAL PHO < >

Duration

1. ____________ (years old)
2. < > __________ (years old)
3. < > __________ (months)

*DUR met for SOCIAL PHO < >

Impairment

1. < > home
2. < > school
3. < > peers

SEP ANX	GEN ANX	OCD
1. <a> <b> 2. <a> <b> 3. < > 4. <a> <b> 5. <a> <b> 6. <a> <b> 7. <a> <b> 8. <a> <b>	1. < > ______________ ______________ ______________ ______________ ______________ 2. <a> <b> 3. <a> <b> <c> <d> <e> <f>	A. Compulsions 1. < > ______________ 2. <a> ______________ <b> 3. < > B. Obsessions 1. <a> ______________ <b> ______________ <c> ______________ 2. <a> <b> <c> 3. < > C. Interference 1. <a> <b> <c>
Criteria If ≥3, then criteria met SEP ANX < >	**Criteria** If 1–3, then criteria met GEN ANX < >	**Criteria** If A1, A2, & C, then criteria met Compulsions < > If B1, B2, & C, then criteria met Obsessions < > If Compulsions + and/or Obsessions +, then criteria met OCD < >
Duration 1. __________ (years old) 2. < > ________ (years old) 3. < > ________ (weeks) *DUR met for SEP ANX < >	**Duration** 1. __________ (years old) 2. < > ________ (years old) 3. < > ________ (months) *DUR met for GEN ANX < >	**Duration** 1. __________ (years old) 2. < > ________ (years old) ________ (months) *DUR met for OCD < >
Impairment 1. < > home 2. < > school 3. < > peers	**Impairment** 1. < > home 2. < > school 3. < > peers	**Impairment** 1. < > home 2. < > school 3. < > peers

STRESS (ASD/PTSD)	ANO	BUL
A. Exposure 1. <a> <b> ____________ 2. <a> <b> <c> <d> <e> 3. < > ____________ B. Dissociation 1. <a> <b> <c> <d> 2. < > 3. < > 4. < > 5. < > C. Reexperiencing 1. <a> <b> <c> 2. <a> <b> 3. <a> <b> 4. <a> <b> 5. < > D. Avoidance 1. <a> <b> 2. <a> <b> <c> 3. < > 4. <a> <b> 5. <a> <b> 6. <a> <b> 7. <a> <b> E. Hyperarousal 1. <a> <b> 2. <a> <b> 3. < > 4. < > 5. < >	1. <a> <b> 2. <a> ht: ____________ wt: ____________ <b> ht: ____________ wt: ____________ 3. <a> <b> <c> 4. <a> <b> <c> 5. < >	1. < > ____________ ____________ 2. <a> <b> <c> <d> 3. <a> <b> <c> <d> 4. <a> <b>
Criteria If A1 & A2, ≥3 in B, ≥1 in C, ≥3 in D, and ≥2 in E, then criteria met ASD < > If A1 & A2, ≥1 in C, ≥3 in D, and ≥2 in E, then criteria met PTSD < >	**Criteria** If 1–4 (&5 for pubescent girls), then criteria met ANO < >	**Criteria** If 1–4, then criteria met BUL < >
Duration 1. ____________ (years old) 2. < > ____________ (years old) 3. a. < > ________ (weeks) b. < > c. < > ________ (days) 4. < > ____________ (months) *DUR met for ASD < > *DUR met for PTSD < >	**Duration** 1. ____________ (years old) 2. < > ________ (years old) 3. < > ________ (months) *DUR met for ANO < >	**Duration** 1. ____________ (years old) 2. < > ________ (years old) 3. a. < > ______ (#/week) b. < > ______ (months) *DUR met for BUL < >
Impairment 1. < > home 2. < > school 3. < > peers **Type (PTSD)** Acute < > Regular Onset < > Chronic < > Delayed Onset < >	**Impairment** 1. < > home 2. < > school 3. < > peers	**Impairment** 1. < > home 2. < > school 3. < > peers

DEP/DYS (MDD/DD)

A. Dysphoric Mood
1. <a> <b> <c>
2. <a> <bi> <bii> <biii> <c> <d>

B. Loss of Interest
1. <a> <b>
2. <a> <b> <c>

C. Appetite Changes
1. <a> <b> <c>
2. <a> <b>

D. Sleep Changes
Bedtime: __________
Wakeup: __________
1. <a> <b> <c>
2. <a> <b>

E. Psychomotor Changes
1. <a> <b> <c> <d>
2. <a> <b>

F. Low Energy
1. <a> <b> <c> <d>

G. Guilt
1. <a> <b> <c> <d>
2. <a> <b>

H. Impaired Concentration
1. <a> <b> <c> <d> <e>
2. < >

I. Hopelessness
1. <a> <b> <c>

J. Morbid/Suicidal Thoughts
1. <a> <b>
2. <a> <b> <c> <d> <e>

____
____
____
____
____

DEP/DYS (MDD/DD)

Criteria

If A &/or B & ≥5 of A–H or J,
then criteria met
MDD < >

If A & ≥2 of C, D, F, G, H, or I,
then criteria met
DD < >

Duration

1. ______________ (years old)
2. < > __________ (years old)
3. MDD < > _______ (weeks)
   DD < > ________ (months)

*DUR met for MDD < >
*DUR met for DD < >

Impairment

1. < > home
2. < > school
3. < > peers

MAN/HYPOMAN

A. Elevated Mood
1. <a> ____________________
   <b> ____________________
   <c> ____________________
2. < > ____________________

B. Other Symptoms
1. <a> ____________________
   <b>
2. <a> <b> <c> __________
3. <a> <b> <c> <d>
4. <a> <b> <c>
5. < >
6. <a> <b> <c> <d> <e>
7. <a> <b> <c> <d>

C. Interference
1. < >
2. < >

Criteria

If A1(a, b, & c) + ≥3 in B + ≥1 in C
or
A2 + ≥4 in B + ≥1 in C,
then criteria met
MAN < >

If A1(a, b, & c) + ≥3 in B +
none in C
or
A2 + ≥4 in B + none in C,
then criteria met
HYPOMAN < >

Duration

1. ______________ (years old)
2. < > ___________ (years old)
3. MAN < > _______ (weeks)
   HYPO < > ______ (days)

*DUR met for MAN < >
*DUR met for HYPOMAN < >

Impairment

1. < > home
2. < > school
3. < > peers

ENU

1. < >
2. <a> <b>
3. <a> <b>

Criteria

If 1, ≥1 in 2, 3a, and 3b,
then criteria met
ENU < >

Duration

1. ____________ (years old)
2. < > _________ (years old)
3. <a> _________ (x/week)
   <b> _________ (months)

*DUR met for ENU < >

Impairment

1. < > home
2. < > school
3. < > peers

Type

Nocturnal	< >
Diurnal	< >
Both	< >

ENC

1. < >
2. < >

Criteria

If both 1 & 2, then criteria met
ENC < >

Duration

1. ____________ (years old)
2. < > _________ (years old)
3. <a> _________ (x/month)
   <b> _________ (months)

*DUR met for ENC < >

Impairment

1. < > home
2. < > school
3. < > peers

SCZ/PSY

A. Psychotic Symptoms
1. <a> <b> <c> <d> <e>
2. <a> <b> <c> <d> <e> <f>
3. < >
4. < >
5. < >

B. Interference
1. < >
2. < >
3. < >

Criteria

If ≥2 in A and ≥1 in B,
then criteria met
SCZ < >

If ≥1 in A, then criteria met
PSY < >

Duration

1. ______________ (years old)
2. < > ___________ (years old)
3. < > ___________ (months)

*DUR met for SCZ < >
*DUR met for PSY < >

Impairment

1. < > home
2. < > school
3. < > peers

STRESSORS

A. Child Abuse/Neglect
1. <a> <b> <c>
2. <a> <b> <c> <d>
3. <a> <b> <c> <d>
4. < >
5. < >

Duration

1. ______________________
2. < > ___________________
3. ______________________
4. ______________________
5. < >

B. Other Stressors
1. <a> <b> <c> <d> <e>
2. < >
3. <a> <b>
4. <a> <b> <c>
5. <a> <b>
6. <a> <b>
7. <a> ________________
   <b>
8. <a> <b> <c> <d>
9. < > ________________
   ____
   ____
10. < >
11. < > ________________
    ____
    ____

P-ChIPS Scoring Form
Profile Sheet

Child's Number: ______________________ Date: ______________
Child's Name: ______________________ Time Started: ______________
Date of Birth: ______________ Age: ______________ Time Ended: ______________
Race: ______________ Sex: ______________ Interviewer: ______________
Informant's Name: ______________________
Informant's Relationship (circle one): Mother, Father, Stepmother, Stepfather, Guardian, Other: ______________

	Disorder	Symptoms	Diagnosis	Duration	Clinician's Diagnosis
ADHD	**Attention-Deficit/Hyperactivity Disorder** *Type:* Inattentive, Hyperactive–Impulsive, Combined	<>	<>	<>	**Axis I**
ODD	**Oppositional Defiant Disorder**	<>	<>	<>	
CD	**Conduct Disorder** *Onset:* Childhood, Adolescent *Severity:* Mild, Moderate, Severe	<>	<>	<>	
SUBAB	**Substance Abuse** *Substance(s):* ______________	<>	<>	<>	
PHO	**Specific Phobia** *Type:* ______________	<>	<>	<>	**Axis II**
SOCPHO	**Social Phobia**	<>	<>	<>	
SEPANX	**Separation Anxiety Disorder**	<>	<>	<>	**Axis III**
GENANX	**General Anxiety Disorder**	<>	<>	<>	
OCD	**Obsessive-Compulsive Disorder**	<>	<>	<>	
PTSD	**Posttraumatic Stress Disorder** *Type:* Acute, Chronic *Onset:* Regular, Delayed	<>	<>	<>	**Axis IV**
ASD	**Acute Stress Disorder**	<>	<>	<>	
ANO	**Anorexia**	<>	<>	<>	**Axis V**
BUL	**Bulimia**	<>	<>	<>	**current:**
DEP	**Major Depressive Disorder**	<>	<>	<>	**past year:**
DYS	**Dysthymic Disorder**	<>	<>	<>	
MAN	**Mania**	<>	<>	<>	
HYPOMAN	**Hypomania**	<>	<>	<>	
ENU	**Enuresis** *Type:* Nocturnal, Diurnal, Both	<>	<>	<>	
ENC	**Encopresis**	<>	<>	<>	
SCZ	**Schizophrenia**	<>	<>	<>	
PSY	**Psychosis**	<>	<>	<>	

Psychosocial Stressors:

Other Stressors:

Behavioral Observations

Appearance:

Affect:

Effort:

Level of Activity:

Unusual Behaviors:

Presenting Problem

Home
1.
2.

School
1.
2.
3.
4.
5.

Peers/Work
1.
2.
3.
4.
5.

Medication
Type:
Dosage:

Child's Name: ______________________________

Date: ________________

ADHD	ODD	CD
A. Inattention 1. <a> <b> 2. < > 3. <a> <b> 4. <a> <b> <c> 5. < > 6. < > 7. < > 8. <a> <b> 9. <a> <b> B. Hyperactivity–Impulsivity 1. <a> <b> 2. <a> <b> 3. < > 4. <a> <b> 5. < > 6. <a> <b> 7. < > 8. <a> <b> 9. <a> <b> <c>	1. <a> <b> 2. <a> <b> 3. <a> <b> <c> <d> 4. < > 5. <a> <b> 6. < > 7. < > 8. < >	1. < > 2. <a> <b> 3. < > 4. < > 5. < > 6. < > 7. <a> <b> 8. <a> <b> 9. < > 10. <a> <b> 11. < > 12. < > 13. < > 14. < > 15. <a> <b>
Criteria If ≥6 in *A only*, then criteria met Inattentive < > If ≥6 in *B only*, then criteria met Hyperactive–Impulsive < > If ≥6 in A *and* ≥6 in B, then criteria met Combined < >	**Criteria** If ≥4, then criteria met ODD < >	**Criteria** If ≥3, then criteria met CD < >
Duration 1. ____________ (years old) 2. < > _________ (years old) 3. < > __________ (months) * DUR met for ADHD < >	**Duration** 1. ____________ (years old) 2. < > _________ (years old) 3. < > __________ (months) * DUR met for ODD < >	**Duration** 1. ____________ (years old) 2. < > _________ (years old) 3. < > __________ (months) * DUR met for CD < >
Impairment 1. < > home 2. < > school 3. < > peers	**Impairment** 1. < > home 2. < > school 3. < > peers	**Impairment** 1. < > home 2. < > school 3. < > peers
		Type Childhood Onset < > Adolescent Onset < > Mild < > Moderate < > Severe < >

SUB AB

1. < >
   <a>____________________
   <b>____________________
   <c>____________________
   ____
2. < > ____________________
3. < > ____________________
4. < > ____________________

Duration

1. ____________ (years old)
2. < > __________ (years old)
   __________ (months)

* DUR met for SUB AB < >

Impairment

1. <a> <b>
2. < >
3. <a> <b>
4. < >

Criteria

If any use (Q1–4) and any impairment (1–4), then criteria met SUB AB < >

Type(s) ____________________
____
____
____

PHO

1. ____________________
   ____
   ____
2. <a> <b>
3. <a> <b>
4. <ai> <aii> <aiii> <aiv> <b>
5. <a> <b>

Criteria

If 1–4, then criteria met
PHO < >

Duration

1. ____________ (years old)
2. < > __________ (years old)
3. < > __________ (months)

* DUR met for PHO < >

Impairment

1. < > home
2. < > school
3. < > peers

Type(s)

Animal	< >
Natural Environment	< >
Blood–Injection–Injury	< >
Situational	< >
Other ________________	< >

SOCIAL PHO

1. <a> <b>
2. < >
3. <a> <b>
4. <ai> <aii> <aiii> <aiv> <b>
5. < >

Criteria

If 1–4, then criteria met
SOCIAL PHO < >

Duration

1. ____________ (years old)
2. < > __________ (years old)
3. < > __________ (months)

*DUR met for SOCIAL PHO < >

Impairment

1. < > home
2. < > school
3. < > peers

SEP ANX	GEN ANX	OCD
1. <a> <b> 2. <a> <b> 3. < > 4. <a> <b> 5. <a> <b> 6. <a> <b> 7. <a> <b> 8. <a> <b>	1. < > ____________ ____________ ____________ ____________ ____________ 2. <a> <b> 3. <a> <b> <c> <d> <e> <f>	A. Compulsions 1. < > ____________ 2. <a> ____________ <b> 3. < > B. Obsessions 1. <a> ____________ <b> ____________ <c> ____________ 2. <a> <b> <c> 3. < > C. Interference 1. <a> <b> <c>
Criteria If ≥3, then criteria met SEP ANX < >	**Criteria** If 1–3, then criteria met GEN ANX < >	**Criteria** If A1, A2, & C, then criteria met Compulsions < > If B1, B2, & C, then criteria met Obsessions < > If Compulsions + and/or Obsessions +, then criteria met OCD < >
Duration 1. ____________ (years old) 2. < > __________ (years old) 3. < > __________ (weeks) *DUR met for SEP ANX < >	**Duration** 1. ____________ (years old) 2. < > __________ (years old) 3. < > __________ (months) *DUR met for GEN ANX < >	**Duration** 1. ____________ (years old) 2. < > __________ (years old) __________ (months) *DUR met for OCD < >
Impairment 1. < > home 2. < > school 3. < > peers	**Impairment** 1. < > home 2. < > school 3. < > peers	**Impairment** 1. < > home 2. < > school 3. < > peers

STRESS (ASD/PTSD)	ANO	BUL
A. Exposure 1. <a> <b> ______________ 2. <a> <b> <c> <d> <e> 3. < > ________________ B. Dissociation 1. <a> <b> <c> <d> 2. < > 3. < > 4. < > 5. < > C. Reexperiencing 1. <a> <b> <c> 2. <a> <b> 3. <a> <b> 4. <a> <b> 5. < > D. Avoidance 1. <a> <b> 2. <a> <b> <c> 3. < > 4. <a> <b> 5. <a> <b> 6. <a> <b> 7. <a> <b> E. Hyperarousal 1. <a> <b> 2. <a> <b> 3. < > 4. < > 5. < >	1. <a> <b> 2. <a> ht: ____________ wt: ____________ <b> ht: ____________ wt: ____________ 3. <a> <b> <c> 4. <a> <b> <c> 5. < >	1. < > ______________ ______________________ 2. <a> <b> <c> <d> 3. <a> <b> <c> <d> 4. <a> <b>
Criteria If A1 & A2, ≥3 in B, ≥1 in C, ≥3 in D, and ≥2 in E, then criteria met ASD < > If A1 & A2, ≥1 in C, ≥3 in D, and ≥2 in E, then criteria met PTSD < >	**Criteria** If 1–4 (&5 for pubescent girls), then criteria met ANO < >	**Criteria** If 1–4, then criteria met BUL < >
Duration 1. __________ (years old) 2. < > ________ (years old) 3. a. < > ______ (weeks) b. < > c. < > ______ (days) 4. < > ________ (months) *DUR met for ASD < > *DUR met for PTSD < >	**Duration** 1. __________ (years old) 2. < > ______ (years old) 3. < > ______ (months) *DUR met for ANO < >	**Duration** 1. __________ (years old) 2. < > ______ (years old) 3. a. < > _____ (#/week) b. < > _____ (months) *DUR met for BUL < >
Impairment 1. < > home 2. < > school 3. < > peers **Type (PTSD)** Acute < > Regular Onset < > Chronic < > Delayed Onset < >	**Impairment** 1. < > home 2. < > school 3. < > peers	**Impairment** 1. < > home 2. < > school 3. < > peers

DEP/DYS (MDD/DD)

A. Dysphoric Mood
1. <a> <b> <c>
2. <a> <bi> <bii> <biii> <c> <d>

B. Loss of Interest
1. <a> <b>
2. <a> <b> <c>

C. Appetite Changes
1. <a> <b> <c>
2. <a> <b>

D. Sleep Changes
Bedtime: __________
Wakeup: __________
1. <a> <b> <c>
2. <a> <b>

E. Psychomotor Changes
1. <a> <b> <c> <d>
2. <a> <b>

F. Low Energy
1. <a> <b> <c> <d>

G. Guilt
1. <a> <b> <c> <d>
2. <a> <b>

H. Impaired Concentration
1. <a> <b> <c> <d> <e>
2. < >

I. Hopelessness
1. <a> <b> <c>

J. Morbid/Suicidal Thoughts
1. <a> <b>
2. <a> <b> <c> <d> <e>

____
____
____
____
____

DEP/DYS (MDD/DD)

Criteria

If A &/or B & ≥5 of A–H or J, then criteria met
MDD < >

If A & ≥2 of C, D, F, G, H, or I, then criteria met
DD < >

Duration
1. ______________ (years old)
2. < > __________ (years old)
3. MDD < > _______ (weeks)
   DD < > ________ (months)

*DUR met for MDD < >
*DUR met for DD < >

Impairment
1. < > home
2. < > school
3. < > peers

MAN/HYPOMAN

A. Elevated Mood
1. <a> ____________________
   <b> ____________________
   <c> ____________________
2. < > ____________________

B. Other Symptoms
1. <a> ____________________
   <b>
2. <a> <b> <c> ____________
3. <a> <b> <c> <d>
4. <a> <b> <c>
5. < >
6. <a> <b> <c> <d> <e>
7. <a> <b> <c> <d>

C. Interference
1. < >
2. < >

Criteria

If A1(a, b, & c) + ≥3 in B + ≥1 in C
or
A2 + ≥4 in B + ≥1 in C, then criteria met
MAN < >

If A1(a, b, & c) + ≥3 in B + none in C
or
A2 + ≥4 in B + none in C, then criteria met
HYPOMAN < >

Duration
1. ______________ (years old)
2. < > ___________ (years old)
3. MAN < > _______ (weeks)
   HYPO < > ______ (days)

*DUR met for MAN < >
*DUR met for HYPOMAN < >

Impairment
1. < > home
2. < > school
3. < > peers

ENU

1. < >
2. <a> <b>
3. <a> <b>

Criteria

If 1, ≥1 in 2, 3a, and 3b, then criteria met

ENU < >

Duration

1. __________ (years old)
2. < > __________ (years old)
3. <a> __________ (x/week)
   <b> __________ (months)

*DUR met for ENU < >

Impairment

1. < > home
2. < > school
3. < > peers

Type

Nocturnal	< >
Diurnal	< >
Both	< >

ENC

1. < >
2. < >

Criteria

If both 1 & 2, then criteria met

ENC < >

Duration

1. __________ (years old)
2. < > __________ (years old)
3. <a> __________ (x/month)
   <b> __________ (months)

*DUR met for ENC < >

Impairment

1. < > home
2. < > school
3. < > peers

SCZ/PSY

A. Psychotic Symptoms

1. <a> <b> <c> <d> <e>
2. <a> <b> <c> <d> <e> <f>
3. < >
4. < >
5. < >

B. Interference

1. < >
2. < >
3. < >

Criteria

If ≥2 in A and ≥1 in B, then criteria met

SCZ < >

If ≥1 in A, then criteria met

PSY < >

Duration

1. __________ (years old)
2. < > __________ (years old)
3. < > __________ (months)

*DUR met for SCZ < >

*DUR met for PSY < >

Impairment

1. < > home
2. < > school
3. < > peers

STRESSORS

A. Child Abuse/Neglect

1. <a> <b> <c>
2. <a> <b> <c> <d>
3. <a> <b> <c> <d>
4. < >
5. < >

Duration

1. __________
2. < > __________
3. __________
4. __________
5. < >

B. Other Stressors

1. <a> <b> <c> <d> <e>
2. < >
3. <a> <b>
4. <a> <b> <c>
5. <a> <b>
6. <a> <b>
7. <a> __________
   <b>
8. <a> <b> <c> <d>
9. < > __________
   ____
   ____
10. < >
11. < > __________
    ____
    ____

P-ChIPS Scoring Form
Profile Sheet

Child's Number: ______________________ Date: ______________

Child's Name: ______________________ Time Started: ______________

Date of Birth: ______________ Age: ______________ Time Ended: ______________

Race: ______________ Sex: ______________ Interviewer: ______________

Informant's Name: ______________________

Informant's Relationship (circle one): Mother, Father, Stepmother, Stepfather, Guardian, Other: ______________

	Disorder	Symptoms	Diagnosis	Duration	Clinician's Diagnosis
ADHD	**Attention-Deficit/Hyperactivity Disorder**	<>	<>	<>	**Axis I**
	Type: Inattentive, Hyperactive–Impulsive, Combined				
ODD	**Oppositional Defiant Disorder**	<>	<>	<>	
CD	**Conduct Disorder**	<>	<>	<>	
	Onset: Childhood, Adolescent				
	Severity: Mild, Moderate, Severe				
SUBAB	**Substance Abuse**	<>	<>	<>	
	Substance(s): ______________				
PHO	**Specific Phobia**	<>	<>	<>	**Axis II**
	Type: ______________				
SOCPHO	**Social Phobia**	<>	<>	<>	
SEPANX	**Separation Anxiety Disorder**	<>	<>	<>	**Axis III**
GENANX	**General Anxiety Disorder**	<>	<>	<>	
OCD	**Obsessive-Compulsive Disorder**	<>	<>	<>	
PTSD	**Posttraumatic Stress Disorder**	<>	<>	<>	**Axis IV**
	Type: Acute, Chronic				
	Onset: Regular, Delayed				
ASD	**Acute Stress Disorder**	<>	<>	<>	
ANO	**Anorexia**	<>	<>	<>	**Axis V**
BUL	**Bulimia**	<>	<>	<>	**current:**
DEP	**Major Depressive Disorder**	<>	<>	<>	**past year:**
DYS	**Dysthymic Disorder**	<>	<>	<>	
MAN	**Mania**	<>	<>	<>	
HYPOMAN	**Hypomania**	<>	<>	<>	
ENU	**Enuresis**	<>	<>	<>	
	Type: Nocturnal, Diurnal, Both				
ENC	**Encopresis**	<>	<>	<>	
SCZ	**Schizophrenia**	<>	<>	<>	
PSY	**Psychosis**	<>	<>	<>	

Psychosocial Stressors:

Other Stressors:

Behavioral Observations

Appearance:

Affect:

Effort:

Level of Activity:

Unusual Behaviors:

Presenting Problem

Home

1.

2.

School

1.

2.

3.

4.

5.

Peers/Work

1.

2.

3.

4.

5.

Medication

Type:

Dosage:

Child's Name: ______________________________

Date: ______________

ADHD	ODD	CD
A. Inattention 1. <a> <b> 2. < > 3. <a> <b> 4. <a> <b> <c> 5. < > 6. < > 7. < > 8. <a> <b> 9. <a> <b> B. Hyperactivity–Impulsivity 1. <a> <b> 2. <a> <b> 3. < > 4. <a> <b> 5. < > 6. <a> <b> 7. < > 8. <a> <b> 9. <a> <b> <c>	1. <a> <b> 2. <a> <b> 3. <a> <b> <c> <d> 4. < > 5. <a> <b> 6. < > 7. < > 8. < >	1. < > 2. <a> <b> 3. < > 4. < > 5. < > 6. < > 7. <a> <b> 8. <a> <b> 9. < > 10. <a> <b> 11. < > 12. < > 13. < > 14. < > 15. <a> <b>
Criteria If $\geq$6 in *A only*, then criteria met Inattentive < > If $\geq$6 in *B only*, then criteria met Hyperactive–Impulsive < > If $\geq$6 in A *and* $\geq$6 in B, then criteria met Combined < >	**Criteria** If $\geq$4, then criteria met ODD < >	**Criteria** If $\geq$3, then criteria met CD < >
Duration 1. ____________ (years old) 2. < > _________ (years old) 3. < > __________ (months) * DUR met for ADHD < >	**Duration** 1. ____________ (years old) 2. < > _________ (years old) 3. < > __________ (months) * DUR met for ODD < >	**Duration** 1. ____________ (years old) 2. < > _________ (years old) 3. < > __________ (months) * DUR met for CD < >
Impairment 1. < > home 2. < > school 3. < > peers	**Impairment** 1. < > home 2. < > school 3. < > peers	**Impairment** 1. < > home 2. < > school 3. < > peers
		Type Childhood Onset < > Adolescent Onset < > Mild < > Moderate < > Severe < >

SUB AB

1. < >
   <a>______
   <b>______
   <c>______
   ______
2. < > ______
3. < > ______
4. < > ______

Duration

1. ______ (years old)
2. < > ______ (years old)
   ______ (months)

* DUR met for SUB AB < >

Impairment

1. <a> <b>
2. < >
3. <a> <b>
4. < >

Criteria

If any use (Q1–4) and any impairment (1–4), then criteria met SUB AB < >

Type(s) ______

______

______

______

PHO

1. ______
   ______
   ______
2. <a> <b>
3. <a> <b>
4. <ai> <aii> <aiii> <aiv> <b>
5. <a> <b>

Criteria

If 1–4, then criteria met PHO < >

Duration

1. ______ (years old)
2. < > ______ (years old)
3. < > ______ (months)

* DUR met for PHO < >

Impairment

1. < > home
2. < > school
3. < > peers

Type(s)

Animal	< >
Natural Environment	< >
Blood–Injection–Injury	< >
Situational	< >
Other ______	< >

SOCIAL PHO

1. <a> <b>
2. < >
3. <a> <b>
4. <ai> <aii> <aiii> <aiv> <b>
5. < >

Criteria

If 1–4, then criteria met SOCIAL PHO < >

Duration

1. ______ (years old)
2. < > ______ (years old)
3. < > ______ (months)

*DUR met for SOCIAL PHO < >

Impairment

1. < > home
2. < > school
3. < > peers

SEP ANX	GEN ANX	OCD
1. <a> <b> 2. <a> <b> 3. < > 4. <a> <b> 5. <a> <b> 6. <a> <b> 7. <a> <b> 8. <a> <b>	1. < > ____________ ____________ ____________ ____________ ____________ 2. <a> <b> 3. <a> <b> <c> <d> <e> <f>	A. Compulsions 1. < > ____________ 2. <a> ____________ <b> 3. < > B. Obsessions 1. <a> ____________ <b> ____________ <c> ____________ 2. <a> <b> <c> 3. < > C. Interference 1. <a> <b> <c>
Criteria If ≥3, then criteria met SEP ANX < >	**Criteria** If 1–3, then criteria met GEN ANX < >	**Criteria** If A1, A2, & C, then criteria met Compulsions < > If B1, B2, & C, then criteria met Obsessions < > If Compulsions + and/or Obsessions +, then criteria met OCD < >
Duration 1. ____________ (years old) 2. < > __________ (years old) 3. < > __________ (weeks) *DUR met for SEP ANX < >	**Duration** 1. ____________ (years old) 2. < > __________ (years old) 3. < > __________ (months) *DUR met for GEN ANX < >	**Duration** 1. ____________ (years old) 2. < > __________ (years old) __________ (months) *DUR met for OCD < >
Impairment 1. < > home 2. < > school 3. < > peers	**Impairment** 1. < > home 2. < > school 3. < > peers	**Impairment** 1. < > home 2. < > school 3. < > peers

STRESS (ASD/PTSD)	ANO	BUL
A. Exposure 1. <a> <b> ________________ 2. <a> <b> <c> <d> <e> 3. < > ____________________ B. Dissociation 1. <a> <b> <c> <d> 2. < > 3. < > 4. < > 5. < > C. Reexperiencing 1. <a> <b> <c> 2. <a> <b> 3. <a> <b> 4. <a> <b> 5. < > D. Avoidance 1. <a> <b> 2. <a> <b> <c> 3. < > 4. <a> <b> 5. <a> <b> 6. <a> <b> 7. <a> <b> E. Hyperarousal 1. <a> <b> 2. <a> <b> 3. < > 4. < > 5. < >	1. <a> <b> 2. <a> ht: ____________ wt: ____________ <b> ht: ____________ wt: ____________ 3. <a> <b> <c> 4. <a> <b> <c> 5. < >	1. < > ________________ ________________________ 2. <a> <b> <c> <d> 3. <a> <b> <c> <d> 4. <a> <b>
Criteria If A1 & A2, $\geq$3 in B, $\geq$1 in C, $\geq$3 in D, and $\geq$2 in E, then criteria met ASD < > If A1 & A2, $\geq$1 in C, $\geq$3 in D, and $\geq$2 in E, then criteria met PTSD < >	**Criteria** If 1–4 (&5 for pubescent girls), then criteria met ANO < >	**Criteria** If 1–4, then criteria met BUL < >
Duration 1. ____________ (years old) 2. < > __________ (years old) 3. a. < > _______ (weeks) b. < > c. < > _______ (days) 4. < > __________ (months) *DUR met for ASD < > *DUR met for PTSD < >	**Duration** 1. __________ (years old) 2. < > _______ (years old) 3. < > _______ (months) *DUR met for ANO < >	**Duration** 1. __________ (years old) 2. < > _______ (years old) 3. a. < > _____ (#/week) b. < > _____ (months) *DUR met for BUL < >
Impairment 1. < > home 2. < > school 3. < > peers **Type (PTSD)** Acute < > Regular Onset < > Chronic < > Delayed Onset < >	**Impairment** 1. < > home 2. < > school 3. < > peers	**Impairment** 1. < > home 2. < > school 3. < > peers

DEP/DYS (MDD/DD)

A. Dysphoric Mood
1. <a> <b> <c>
2. <a> <bi> <bii> <biii> <c> <d>

B. Loss of Interest
1. <a> <b>
2. <a> <b> <c>

C. Appetite Changes
1. <a> <b> <c>
2. <a> <b>

D. Sleep Changes
Bedtime: __________
Wakeup: __________
1. <a> <b> <c>
2. <a> <b>

E. Psychomotor Changes
1. <a> <b> <c> <d>
2. <a> <b>

F. Low Energy
1. <a> <b> <c> <d>

G. Guilt
1. <a> <b> <c> <d>
2. <a> <b>

H. Impaired Concentration
1. <a> <b> <c> <d> <e>
2. < >

I. Hopelessness
1. <a> <b> <c>

J. Morbid/Suicidal Thoughts
1. <a> <b>
2. <a> <b> <c> <d> <e>

____
____
____
____
____

DEP/DYS (MDD/DD)

Criteria

If A &/or B & ≥5 of A–H or J, then criteria met
MDD < >

If A & ≥2 of C, D, F, G, H, or I, then criteria met
DD < >

Duration

1. ______________ (years old)
2. < > ______________ (years old)
3. MDD < > ________ (weeks)
   DD < > ________ (months)

*DUR met for MDD < >
*DUR met for DD < >

Impairment

1. < > home
2. < > school
3. < > peers

MAN/HYPOMAN

A. Elevated Mood
1. <a> ____________________
   <b> ____________________
   <c> ____________________
2. < > ____________________

B. Other Symptoms
1. <a> ____________________
   <b>
2. <a> <b> <c> ____________
3. <a> <b> <c> <d>
4. <a> <b> <c>
5. < >
6. <a> <b> <c> <d> <e>
7. <a> <b> <c> <d>

C. Interference
1. < >
2. < >

Criteria

If A1(a, b, & c) + ≥3 in B + ≥1 in C
or
A2 + ≥4 in B + ≥1 in C, then criteria met
MAN < >

If A1(a, b, & c) + ≥3 in B + none in C
or
A2 + ≥4 in B + none in C, then criteria met
HYPOMAN < >

Duration

1. ______________ (years old)
2. < > ______________ (years old)
3. MAN < > ________ (weeks)
   HYPO < > ________ (days)

*DUR met for MAN < >
*DUR met for HYPOMAN < >

Impairment

1. < > home
2. < > school
3. < > peers

ENU

1. < >
2. <a> <b>
3. <a> <b>

Criteria

If 1, ≥1 in 2, 3a, and 3b, then criteria met
ENU < >

Duration

1. ____________ (years old)
2. < > ________ (years old)
3. <a> ________ (x/week)
   <b> ________ (months)

*DUR met for ENU < >

Impairment

1. < > home
2. < > school
3. < > peers

Type

Nocturnal	< >
Diurnal	< >
Both	< >

ENC

1. < >
2. < >

Criteria

If both 1 & 2, then criteria met
ENC < >

Duration

1. ____________ (years old)
2. < > ________ (years old)
3. <a> ________ (x/month)
   <b> ________ (months)

*DUR met for ENC < >

Impairment

1. < > home
2. < > school
3. < > peers

SCZ/PSY

A. Psychotic Symptoms
1. <a> <b> <c> <d> <e>
2. <a> <b> <c> <d> <e> <f>
3. < >
4. < >
5. < >

B. Interference
1. < >
2. < >
3. < >

Criteria

If ≥2 in A and ≥1 in B, then criteria met
SCZ < >

If ≥1 in A, then criteria met
PSY < >

Duration

1. ____________ (years old)
2. < > __________ (years old)
3. < > __________ (months)

*DUR met for SCZ < >
*DUR met for PSY < >

Impairment

1. < > home
2. < > school
3. < > peers

STRESSORS

A. Child Abuse/Neglect
1. <a> <b> <c>
2. <a> <b> <c> <d>
3. <a> <b> <c> <d>
4. < >
5. < >

Duration

1. ____________________
2. < > ________________
3. ____________________
4. ____________________
5. < >

B. Other Stressors
1. <a> <b> <c> <d> <e>
2. < >
3. <a> <b>
4. <a> <b> <c>
5. <a> <b>
6. <a> <b>
7. <a> ______________
   <b>
8. <a> <b> <c> <d>
9. < > ______________
   ____
   ____
10. < >
11. < > ______________
    ____
    ____

P-ChIPS Scoring Form
Profile Sheet

Child's Number: ______________________ Date: ______________

Child's Name: ______________________ Time Started: ______________

Date of Birth: ______________ Age: ______________ Time Ended: ______________

Race: ______________ Sex: ______________ Interviewer: ______________

Informant's Name: ______________________

Informant's Relationship (circle one): Mother, Father, Stepmother, Stepfather, Guardian, Other: ______________

	Disorder	Symptoms	Diagnosis	Duration	Clinician's Diagnosis
ADHD	**Attention-Deficit/Hyperactivity Disorder** *Type:* Inattentive, Hyperactive–Impulsive, Combined	<>	<>	<>	**Axis I**
ODD	**Oppositional Defiant Disorder**	<>	<>	<>	
CD	**Conduct Disorder** *Onset:* Childhood, Adolescent *Severity:* Mild, Moderate, Severe	<>	<>	<>	
SUBAB	**Substance Abuse** *Substance(s):* ____________	<>	<>	<>	
PHO	**Specific Phobia** *Type:* ____________	<>	<>	<>	**Axis II**
SOCPHO	**Social Phobia**	<>	<>	<>	
SEPANX	**Separation Anxiety Disorder**	<>	<>	<>	**Axis III**
GENANX	**General Anxiety Disorder**	<>	<>	<>	
OCD	**Obsessive-Compulsive Disorder**	<>	<>	<>	
PTSD	**Posttraumatic Stress Disorder** *Type:* Acute, Chronic *Onset:* Regular, Delayed	<>	<>	<>	**Axis IV**
ASD	**Acute Stress Disorder**	<>	<>	<>	
ANO	**Anorexia**	<>	<>	<>	**Axis V**
BUL	**Bulimia**	<>	<>	<>	**current:**
DEP	**Major Depressive Disorder**	<>	<>	<>	**past year:**
DYS	**Dysthymic Disorder**	<>	<>	<>	
MAN	**Mania**	<>	<>	<>	
HYPOMAN	**Hypomania**	<>	<>	<>	
ENU	**Enuresis** *Type:* Nocturnal, Diurnal, Both	<>	<>	<>	
ENC	**Encopresis**	<>	<>	<>	
SCZ	**Schizophrenia**	<>	<>	<>	
PSY	**Psychosis**	<>	<>	<>	

Psychosocial Stressors:

Other Stressors:

Behavioral Observations

Appearance:

Affect:

Effort:

Level of Activity:

Unusual Behaviors:

Presenting Problem

Home

1.

2.

School

1.

2.

3.

4.

5.

Peers/Work

1.

2.

3.

4.

5.

Medication

Type:

Dosage:

Child's Name: ______________________________

Date: ______________

ADHD	ODD	CD
A. Inattention 1. <a> <b> 2. < > 3. <a> <b> 4. <a> <b> <c> 5. < > 6. < > 7. < > 8. <a> <b> 9. <a> <b> B. Hyperactivity–Impulsivity 1. <a> <b> 2. <a> <b> 3. < > 4. <a> <b> 5. < > 6. <a> <b> 7. < > 8. <a> <b> 9. <a> <b> <c>	1. <a> <b> 2. <a> <b> 3. <a> <b> <c> <d> 4. < > 5. <a> <b> 6. < > 7. < > 8. < >	1. < > 2. <a> <b> 3. < > 4. < > 5. < > 6. < > 7. <a> <b> 8. <a> <b> 9. < > 10. <a> <b> 11. < > 12. < > 13. < > 14. < > 15. <a> <b>
Criteria If ≥6 in *A only*, then criteria met Inattentive < > If ≥6 in *B only*, then criteria met Hyperactive–Impulsive < > If ≥6 in A *and* ≥6 in B, then criteria met Combined < >	**Criteria** If ≥4, then criteria met ODD < >	**Criteria** If ≥3, then criteria met CD < >
Duration 1. __________ (years old) 2. < > ________ (years old) 3. < > ________ (months) * DUR met for ADHD < >	**Duration** 1. __________ (years old) 2. < > ________ (years old) 3. < > ________ (months) * DUR met for ODD < >	**Duration** 1. __________ (years old) 2. < > ________ (years old) 3. < > ________ (months) * DUR met for CD < >
Impairment 1. < > home 2. < > school 3. < > peers	**Impairment** 1. < > home 2. < > school 3. < > peers	**Impairment** 1. < > home 2. < > school 3. < > peers **Type** Childhood Onset < > Adolescent Onset < > Mild < > Moderate < > Severe < >

SUB AB

1. < >
   <a>____________________
   <b>____________________
   <c>____________________
   ____
2. < > ____________________
3. < > ____________________
4. < > ____________________

Duration

1. __________ (years old)
2. < > __________ (years old)
   __________ (months)

* DUR met for SUB AB < >

Impairment

1. <a> <b>
2. < >
3. <a> <b>
4. < >

Criteria

If any use (Q1–4) and any impairment (1–4), then criteria met SUB AB < >

Type(s) ____________________

____

____

____

PHO

1. ____________________
   ____
   ____
2. <a> <b>
3. <a> <b>
4. <ai> <aii> <aiii> <aiv> <b>
5. <a> <b>

Criteria

If 1–4, then criteria met PHO < >

Duration

1. __________ (years old)
2. < > __________ (years old)
3. < > __________ (months)

* DUR met for PHO < >

Impairment

1. < > home
2. < > school
3. < > peers

Type(s)

Animal	< >
Natural Environment	< >
Blood–Injection–Injury	< >
Situational	< >
Other ______________	< >

SOCIAL PHO

1. <a> <b>
2. < >
3. <a> <b>
4. <ai> <aii> <aiii> <aiv> <b>
5. < >

Criteria

If 1–4, then criteria met SOCIAL PHO < >

Duration

1. __________ (years old)
2. < > __________ (years old)
3. < > __________ (months)

*DUR met for SOCIAL PHO < >

Impairment

1. < > home
2. < > school
3. < > peers

SEP ANX	GEN ANX	OCD
1. <a> <b> 2. <a> <b> 3. < > 4. <a> <b> 5. <a> <b> 6. <a> <b> 7. <a> <b> 8. <a> <b>	1. < > ____________ ____________ ____________ ____________ ____________ 2. <a> <b> 3. <a> <b> <c> <d> <e> <f>	A. Compulsions 1. < > ____________ 2. <a> ____________ <b> 3. < > B. Obsessions 1. <a> ____________ <b> ____________ <c> ____________ 2. <a> <b> <c> 3. < > C. Interference 1. <a> <b> <c>
Criteria If ≥3, then criteria met SEP ANX < >	**Criteria** If 1–3, then criteria met GEN ANX < >	**Criteria** If A1, A2, & C, then criteria met Compulsions < > If B1, B2, & C, then criteria met Obsessions < > If Compulsions + and/or Obsessions +, then criteria met OCD < >
Duration 1. ____________ (years old) 2. < > __________ (years old) 3. < > __________ (weeks) *DUR met for SEP ANX < >	**Duration** 1. ____________ (years old) 2. < > __________ (years old) 3. < > __________ (months) *DUR met for GEN ANX < >	**Duration** 1. ____________ (years old) 2. < > __________ (years old) __________ (months) *DUR met for OCD < >
Impairment 1. < > home 2. < > school 3. < > peers	**Impairment** 1. < > home 2. < > school 3. < > peers	**Impairment** 1. < > home 2. < > school 3. < > peers

STRESS (ASD/PTSD)	ANO	BUL
A. Exposure 1. <a> <b> ________________ 2. <a> <b> <c> <d> <e> 3. < > ______________________ B. Dissociation 1. <a> <b> <c> <d> 2. < > 3. < > 4. < > 5. < > C. Reexperiencing 1. <a> <b> <c> 2. <a> <b> 3. <a> <b> 4. <a> <b> 5. < > D. Avoidance 1. <a> <b> 2. <a> <b> <c> 3. < > 4. <a> <b> 5. <a> <b> 6. <a> <b> 7. <a> <b> E. Hyperarousal 1. <a> <b> 2. <a> <b> 3. < > 4. < > 5. < >	1. <a> <b> 2. <a> ht: ____________ wt: ____________ <b> ht: ____________ wt: ____________ 3. <a> <b> <c> 4. <a> <b> <c> 5. < >	1. < > ________________ ________________________ 2. <a> <b> <c> <d> 3. <a> <b> <c> <d> 4. <a> <b>
Criteria If A1 & A2, ≥3 in B, ≥1 in C, ≥3 in D, and ≥2 in E, then criteria met ASD < > If A1 & A2, ≥1 in C, ≥3 in D, and ≥2 in E, then criteria met PTSD < >	**Criteria** If 1–4 (&5 for pubescent girls), then criteria met ANO < >	**Criteria** If 1–4, then criteria met BUL < >
Duration 1. ____________ (years old) 2. < > __________ (years old) 3. a. < > _______ (weeks) b. < > c. < > _______ (days) 4. < > __________ (months) *DUR met for ASD < > *DUR met for PTSD < >	**Duration** 1. __________ (years old) 2. < > _______ (years old) 3. < > _______ (months) *DUR met for ANO < >	**Duration** 1. __________ (years old) 2. < > _______ (years old) 3. a. < > _____ (#/week) b. < > _____ (months) *DUR met for BUL < >
Impairment 1. < > home 2. < > school 3. < > peers **Type (PTSD)** Acute < > Regular Onset < > Chronic < > Delayed Onset < >	**Impairment** 1. < > home 2. < > school 3. < > peers	**Impairment** 1. < > home 2. < > school 3. < > peers

DEP/DYS (MDD/DD)

A. Dysphoric Mood
1. <a> <b> <c>
2. <a> <bi> <bii> <biii> <c> <d>

B. Loss of Interest
1. <a> <b>
2. <a> <b> <c>

C. Appetite Changes
1. <a> <b> <c>
2. <a> <b>

D. Sleep Changes
Bedtime: __________
Wakeup: __________
1. <a> <b> <c>
2. <a> <b>

E. Psychomotor Changes
1. <a> <b> <c> <d>
2. <a> <b>

F. Low Energy
1. <a> <b> <c> <d>

G. Guilt
1. <a> <b> <c> <d>
2. <a> <b>

H. Impaired Concentration
1. <a> <b> <c> <d> <e>
2. < >

I. Hopelessness
1. <a> <b> <c>

J. Morbid/Suicidal Thoughts
1. <a> <b>
2. <a> <b> <c> <d> <e>

____
____
____
____
____

DEP/DYS (MDD/DD)

Criteria

If A &/or B & ≥5 of A–H or J,
then criteria met
MDD < >

If A & ≥2 of C, D, F, G, H, or I,
then criteria met
DD < >

Duration
1. ______________ (years old)
2. < > ______________ (years old)
3. MDD < > ________ (weeks)
   DD < > ________ (months)

*DUR met for MDD < >
*DUR met for DD < >

Impairment
1. < > home
2. < > school
3. < > peers

MAN/HYPOMAN

A. Elevated Mood
1. <a> ____________________
   <b> ____________________
   <c> ____________________
2. < > ____________________

B. Other Symptoms
1. <a> ____________________
   <b>
2. <a> <b> <c> ____________
3. <a> <b> <c> <d>
4. <a> <b> <c>
5. < >
6. <a> <b> <c> <d> <e>
7. <a> <b> <c> <d>

C. Interference
1. < >
2. < >

Criteria

If A1(a, b, & c) + ≥3 in B + ≥1 in C
or
A2 + ≥4 in B + ≥1 in C,
then criteria met
MAN < >

If A1(a, b, & c) + ≥3 in B + none in C
or
A2 + ≥4 in B + none in C,
then criteria met
HYPOMAN < >

Duration
1. ______________ (years old)
2. < > ______________ (years old)
3. MAN < > ________ (weeks)
   HYPO < > ________ (days)

*DUR met for MAN < >
*DUR met for HYPOMAN < >

Impairment
1. < > home
2. < > school
3. < > peers

ENU

1. < >
2. <a> <b>
3. <a> <b>

Criteria

If 1, ≥1 in 2, 3a, and 3b, then criteria met

ENU < >

Duration

1. ____________ (years old)
2. < > ________ (years old)
3. <a> ________ (x/week)
   <b> ________ (months)

*DUR met for ENU < >

Impairment

1. < > home
2. < > school
3. < > peers

Type

Nocturnal	< >
Diurnal	< >
Both	< >

ENC

1. < >
2. < >

Criteria

If both 1 & 2, then criteria met

ENC < >

Duration

1. ____________ (years old)
2. < > ________ (years old)
3. <a> ________ (x/month)
   <b> ________ (months)

*DUR met for ENC < >

Impairment

1. < > home
2. < > school
3. < > peers

SCZ/PSY

A. Psychotic Symptoms

1. <a> <b> <c> <d> <e>
2. <a> <b> <c> <d> <e> <f>
3. < >
4. < >
5. < >

B. Interference

1. < >
2. < >
3. < >

Criteria

If ≥2 in A and ≥1 in B, then criteria met

SCZ < >

If ≥1 in A, then criteria met

PSY < >

Duration

1. ______________ (years old)
2. < > __________ (years old)
3. < > __________ (months)

*DUR met for SCZ < >

*DUR met for PSY < >

Impairment

1. < > home
2. < > school
3. < > peers

STRESSORS

A. Child Abuse/Neglect

1. <a> <b> <c>
2. <a> <b> <c> <d>
3. <a> <b> <c> <d>
4. < >
5. < >

Duration

1. ______________________
2. < > ____________________
3. ______________________
4. ______________________
5. < >

B. Other Stressors

1. <a> <b> <c> <d> <e>
2. < >
3. <a> <b>
4. <a> <b> <c>
5. <a> <b>
6. <a> <b>
7. <a> ________________
   <b>
8. <a> <b> <c> <d>
9. < > ________________
   ____
   ____
10. < >
11. < > ________________
    ____
    ____

P-ChIPS Scoring Form
Profile Sheet

Child's Number: ____________________ Date: ____________

Child's Name: ____________________ Time Started: ____________

Date of Birth: ____________ Age: ____________ Time Ended: ____________

Race: ____________ Sex: ____________ Interviewer: ____________

Informant's Name: ____________________

Informant's Relationship (circle one): Mother, Father, Stepmother, Stepfather, Guardian, Other: ____________

	Disorder	Symptoms	Diagnosis	Duration	Clinician's Diagnosis
ADHD	**Attention-Deficit/Hyperactivity Disorder** *Type:* Inattentive, Hyperactive–Impulsive, Combined	<>	<>	<>	**Axis I**
ODD	**Oppositional Defiant Disorder**	<>	<>	<>	
CD	**Conduct Disorder** *Onset:* Childhood, Adolescent *Severity:* Mild, Moderate, Severe	<>	<>	<>	
SUBAB	**Substance Abuse** *Substance(s):* ____________	<>	<>	<>	
PHO	**Specific Phobia** *Type:* ____________	<>	<>	<>	**Axis II**
SOCPHO	**Social Phobia**	<>	<>	<>	
SEPANX	**Separation Anxiety Disorder**	<>	<>	<>	**Axis III**
GENANX	**General Anxiety Disorder**	<>	<>	<>	
OCD	**Obsessive-Compulsive Disorder**	<>	<>	<>	
PTSD	**Posttraumatic Stress Disorder** *Type:* Acute, Chronic *Onset:* Regular, Delayed	<>	<>	<>	**Axis IV**
ASD	**Acute Stress Disorder**	<>	<>	<>	
ANO	**Anorexia**	<>	<>	<>	**Axis V**
BUL	**Bulimia**	<>	<>	<>	**current:**
DEP	**Major Depressive Disorder**	<>	<>	<>	**past year:**
DYS	**Dysthymic Disorder**	<>	<>	<>	
MAN	**Mania**	<>	<>	<>	
HYPOMAN	**Hypomania**	<>	<>	<>	
ENU	**Enuresis** *Type:* Nocturnal, Diurnal, Both	<>	<>	<>	
ENC	**Encopresis**	<>	<>	<>	
SCZ	**Schizophrenia**	<>	<>	<>	
PSY	**Psychosis**	<>	<>	<>	

Psychosocial Stressors:

Other Stressors:

Behavioral Observations

Appearance:

Affect:

Effort:

Level of Activity:

Unusual Behaviors:

Presenting Problem

Home

1.

2.

School

1.

2.

3.

4.

5.

Peers/Work

1.

2.

3.

4.

5.

Medication

Type:

Dosage:

Child's Name: ______________________________

Date: ________________

ADHD	ODD	CD
A. Inattention 1. <a> <b> 2. < > 3. <a> <b> 4. <a> <b> <c> 5. < > 6. < > 7. < > 8. <a> <b> 9. <a> <b> B. Hyperactivity–Impulsivity 1. <a> <b> 2. <a> <b> 3. < > 4. <a> <b> 5. < > 6. <a> <b> 7. < > 8. <a> <b> 9. <a> <b> <c>	1. <a> <b> 2. <a> <b> 3. <a> <b> <c> <d> 4. < > 5. <a> <b> 6. < > 7. < > 8. < >	1. < > 2. <a> <b> 3. < > 4. < > 5. < > 6. < > 7. <a> <b> 8. <a> <b> 9. < > 10. <a> <b> 11. < > 12. < > 13. < > 14. < > 15. <a> <b>
Criteria If ≥6 in *A only*, then criteria met Inattentive < > If ≥6 in *B only*, then criteria met Hyperactive–Impulsive < > If ≥6 in A *and* ≥6 in B, then criteria met Combined < >	**Criteria** If ≥4, then criteria met ODD < >	**Criteria** If ≥3, then criteria met CD < >
Duration 1. ____________ (years old) 2. < > _________ (years old) 3. < > __________ (months) * DUR met for ADHD < >	**Duration** 1. ____________ (years old) 2. < > _________ (years old) 3. < > __________ (months) * DUR met for ODD < >	**Duration** 1. ____________ (years old) 2. < > _________ (years old) 3. < > __________ (months) * DUR met for CD < >
Impairment 1. < > home 2. < > school 3. < > peers	**Impairment** 1. < > home 2. < > school 3. < > peers	**Impairment** 1. < > home 2. < > school 3. < > peers **Type** Childhood Onset < > Adolescent Onset < > Mild < > Moderate < > Severe < >

SUB AB

1. < >
   <a>____________________
   <b>____________________
   <c>____________________
   ____
2. < > ____________________
3. < > ____________________
4. < > ____________________

Duration

1. ____________ (years old)
2. < > __________ (years old)
   __________ (months)

* DUR met for SUB AB < >

Impairment

1. <a> <b>
2. < >
3. <a> <b>
4. < >

Criteria

If any use (Q1–4) and any impairment (1–4), then criteria met SUB AB < >

Type(s) ____________________
____
____
____

PHO

1. ____________________
   ____
   ____
2. <a> <b>
3. <a> <b>
4. <ai> <aii> <aiii> <aiv> <b>
5. <a> <b>

Criteria

If 1–4, then criteria met PHO < >

Duration

1. ____________ (years old)
2. < > __________ (years old)
3. < > __________ (months)

* DUR met for PHO < >

Impairment

1. < > home
2. < > school
3. < > peers

Type(s)

Animal	< >
Natural Environment	< >
Blood–Injection–Injury	< >
Situational	< >
Other ________________	< >

SOCIAL PHO

1. <a> <b>
2. < >
3. <a> <b>
4. <ai> <aii> <aiii> <aiv> <b>
5. < >

Criteria

If 1–4, then criteria met SOCIAL PHO < >

Duration

1. ____________ (years old)
2. < > __________ (years old)
3. < > __________ (months)

*DUR met for SOCIAL PHO < >

Impairment

1. < > home
2. < > school
3. < > peers

SEP ANX	GEN ANX	OCD
1. <a> <b> 2. <a> <b> 3. < > 4. <a> <b> 5. <a> <b> 6. <a> <b> 7. <a> <b> 8. <a> <b>	1. < > ______________ ______________ ______________ ______________ ______________ 2. <a> <b> 3. <a> <b> <c> <d> <e> <f>	A. Compulsions 1. < > ______________ 2. <a> ______________ <b> 3. < > B. Obsessions 1. <a> ______________ <b> ______________ <c> ______________ 2. <a> <b> <c> 3. < > C. Interference 1. <a> <b> <c>
Criteria If ≥3, then criteria met SEP ANX < >	**Criteria** If 1–3, then criteria met GEN ANX < >	**Criteria** If A1, A2, & C, then criteria met Compulsions < > If B1, B2, & C, then criteria met Obsessions < > If Compulsions + and/or Obsessions +, then criteria met OCD < >
Duration 1. __________ (years old) 2. < > __________ (years old) 3. < > __________ (weeks) *DUR met for SEP ANX < >	**Duration** 1. __________ (years old) 2. < > __________ (years old) 3. < > __________ (months) *DUR met for GEN ANX < >	**Duration** 1. __________ (years old) 2. < > __________ (years old) __________ (months) *DUR met for OCD < >
Impairment 1. < > home 2. < > school 3. < > peers	**Impairment** 1. < > home 2. < > school 3. < > peers	**Impairment** 1. < > home 2. < > school 3. < > peers

STRESS (ASD/PTSD)	ANO	BUL
A. Exposure 1. <a> <b> ____________ 2. <a> <b> <c> <d> <e> 3. < > ______________ B. Dissociation 1. <a> <b> <c> <d> 2. < > 3. < > 4. < > 5. < > C. Reexperiencing 1. <a> <b> <c> 2. <a> <b> 3. <a> <b> 4. <a> <b> 5. < > D. Avoidance 1. <a> <b> 2. <a> <b> <c> 3. < > 4. <a> <b> 5. <a> <b> 6. <a> <b> 7. <a> <b> E. Hyperarousal 1. <a> <b> 2. <a> <b> 3. < > 4. < > 5. < >	1. <a> <b> 2. <a> ht: __________ wt: __________ <b> ht: __________ wt: __________ 3. <a> <b> <c> 4. <a> <b> <c> 5. < >	1. < > ______________ ______________________ 2. <a> <b> <c> <d> 3. <a> <b> <c> <d> 4. <a> <b>
Criteria If A1 & A2, ≥3 in B, ≥1 in C, ≥3 in D, and ≥2 in E, then criteria met ASD < > If A1 & A2, ≥1 in C, ≥3 in D, and ≥2 in E, then criteria met PTSD < >	**Criteria** If 1–4 (&5 for pubescent girls), then criteria met ANO < >	**Criteria** If 1–4, then criteria met BUL < >
Duration 1. __________ (years old) 2. < > ________ (years old) 3. a. < > ______ (weeks) b. < > c. < > ______ (days) 4. < > ________ (months) *DUR met for ASD < > *DUR met for PTSD < >	**Duration** 1. ________ (years old) 2. < > ______ (years old) 3. < > ______ (months) *DUR met for ANO < >	**Duration** 1. ________ (years old) 2. < > ______ (years old) 3. a. < > _____ (#/week) b. < > _____ (months) *DUR met for BUL < >
Impairment 1. < > home 2. < > school 3. < > peers **Type (PTSD)** Acute < > Regular Onset < > Chronic < > Delayed Onset < >	**Impairment** 1. < > home 2. < > school 3. < > peers	**Impairment** 1. < > home 2. < > school 3. < > peers

DEP/DYS (MDD/DD)

A. Dysphoric Mood
  1. <a> <b> <c>
  2. <a> <bi> <bii> <biii> <c> <d>

B. Loss of Interest
  1. <a> <b>
  2. <a> <b> <c>

C. Appetite Changes
  1. <a> <b> <c>
  2. <a> <b>

D. Sleep Changes
  Bedtime: __________
  Wakeup: __________
  1. <a> <b> <c>
  2. <a> <b>

E. Psychomotor Changes
  1. <a> <b> <c> <d>
  2. <a> <b>

F. Low Energy
  1. <a> <b> <c> <d>

G. Guilt
  1. <a> <b> <c> <d>
  2. <a> <b>

H. Impaired Concentration
  1. <a> <b> <c> <d> <e>
  2. < >

I. Hopelessness
  1. <a> <b> <c>

J. Morbid/Suicidal Thoughts
  1. <a> <b>
  2. <a> <b> <c> <d> <e>

____
____
____
____
____

DEP/DYS (MDD/DD)

Criteria

If A &/or B & ≥5 of A–H or J,
then criteria met
MDD < >

If A & ≥2 of C, D, F, G, H, or I,
then criteria met
DD < >

Duration

1. ______________ (years old)
2. < > ______________ (years old)
3. MDD < > ________ (weeks)
   DD < > ________ (months)

*DUR met for MDD < >
*DUR met for DD < >

Impairment

1. < > home
2. < > school
3. < > peers

MAN/HYPOMAN

A. Elevated Mood
  1. <a> ______________
     <b> ______________
     <c> ______________
  2. < > ______________

B. Other Symptoms
  1. <a> ______________
     <b>
  2. <a> <b> <c> __________
  3. <a> <b> <c> <d>
  4. <a> <b> <c>
  5. < >
  6. <a> <b> <c> <d> <e>
  7. <a> <b> <c> <d>

C. Interference
  1. < >
  2. < >

Criteria

If A1(a, b, & c) + ≥3 in B + ≥1 in C
or
A2 + ≥4 in B + ≥1 in C,
then criteria met
MAN < >

If A1(a, b, & c) + ≥3 in B +
none in C
or
A2 + ≥4 in B + none in C,
then criteria met
HYPOMAN < >

Duration

1. ______________ (years old)
2. < > ______________ (years old)
3. MAN < > ________ (weeks)
   HYPO < > ________ (days)

*DUR met for MAN < >
*DUR met for HYPOMAN < >

Impairment

1. < > home
2. < > school
3. < > peers

ENU

1. < >
2. <a> <b>
3. <a> <b>

Criteria

If 1, ≥1 in 2, 3a, and 3b,
then criteria met
ENU < >

Duration

1. __________ (years old)
2. < > ________ (years old)
3. <a> ________ (x/week)
   <b> ________ (months)

*DUR met for ENU < >

Impairment

1. < > home
2. < > school
3. < > peers

Type

Nocturnal	< >
Diurnal	< >
Both	< >

ENC

1. < >
2. < >

Criteria

If both 1 & 2, then criteria met
ENC < >

Duration

1. __________ (years old)
2. < > ________ (years old)
3. <a> ________ (x/month)
   <b> ________ (months)

*DUR met for ENC < >

Impairment

1. < > home
2. < > school
3. < > peers

SCZ/PSY

A. Psychotic Symptoms
1. <a> <b> <c> <d> <e>
2. <a> <b> <c> <d> <e> <f>
3. < >
4. < >
5. < >

B. Interference
1. < >
2. < >
3. < >

Criteria

If ≥2 in A and ≥1 in B,
then criteria met
SCZ < >

If ≥1 in A, then criteria met
PSY < >

Duration

1. __________ (years old)
2. < > ________ (years old)
3. < > ________ (months)

*DUR met for SCZ < >
*DUR met for PSY < >

Impairment

1. < > home
2. < > school
3. < > peers

STRESSORS

A. Child Abuse/Neglect
1. <a> <b> <c>
2. <a> <b> <c> <d>
3. <a> <b> <c> <d>
4. < >
5. < >

Duration

1. ____________________
2. < > ________________
3. ____________________
4. ____________________
5. < >

B. Other Stressors
1. <a> <b> <c> <d> <e>
2. < >
3. <a> <b>
4. <a> <b> <c>
5. <a> <b>
6. <a> <b>
7. <a> ______________
   <b>
8. <a> <b> <c> <d>
9. < > ______________
   ____
   ____
10. < >
11. < > ______________
    ____
    ____

P-ChIPS Scoring Form
Profile Sheet

Child's Number: ______________________ Date: ______________

Child's Name: ______________________ Time Started: ______________

Date of Birth: ______________ Age: ______________ Time Ended: ______________

Race: ______________ Sex: ______________ Interviewer: ______________

Informant's Name: ______________________

Informant's Relationship (circle one): Mother, Father, Stepmother, Stepfather, Guardian, Other: ______________

Disorder		Symptoms	Diagnosis	Duration	Clinician's Diagnosis
ADHD	**Attention-Deficit/Hyperactivity Disorder** *Type:* Inattentive, Hyperactive–Impulsive, Combined	<>	<>	<>	**Axis I**
ODD	**Oppositional Defiant Disorder**	<>	<>	<>	
CD	**Conduct Disorder** *Onset:* Childhood, Adolescent *Severity:* Mild, Moderate, Severe	<>	<>	<>	
SUBAB	**Substance Abuse** *Substance(s):* ______________	<>	<>	<>	
PHO	**Specific Phobia** *Type:* ______________	<>	<>	<>	**Axis II**
SOCPHO	**Social Phobia**	<>	<>	<>	
SEPANX	**Separation Anxiety Disorder**	<>	<>	<>	**Axis III**
GENANX	**General Anxiety Disorder**	<>	<>	<>	
OCD	**Obsessive-Compulsive Disorder**	<>	<>	<>	
PTSD	**Posttraumatic Stress Disorder** *Type:* Acute, Chronic *Onset:* Regular, Delayed	<>	<>	<>	**Axis IV**
ASD	**Acute Stress Disorder**	<>	<>	<>	
ANO	**Anorexia**	<>	<>	<>	**Axis V** **current:** **past year:**
BUL	**Bulimia**	<>	<>	<>	
DEP	**Major Depressive Disorder**	<>	<>	<>	
DYS	**Dysthymic Disorder**	<>	<>	<>	
MAN	**Mania**	<>	<>	<>	
HYPOMAN	**Hypomania**	<>	<>	<>	
ENU	**Enuresis** *Type:* Nocturnal, Diurnal, Both	<>	<>	<>	
ENC	**Encopresis**	<>	<>	<>	
SCZ	**Schizophrenia**	<>	<>	<>	
PSY	**Psychosis**	<>	<>	<>	

Psychosocial Stressors:

Other Stressors:

Behavioral Observations

Appearance:

Affect:

Effort:

Level of Activity:

Unusual Behaviors:

Presenting Problem

Home

1.

2.

School

1.

2.

3.

4.

5.

Peers/Work

1.

2.

3.

4.

5.

Medication

Type:

Dosage:

Child's Name: ______________________________

Date: ______________

ADHD	ODD	CD
A. Inattention 1. <a> <b> 2. < > 3. <a> <b> 4. <a> <b> <c> 5. < > 6. < > 7. < > 8. <a> <b> 9. <a> <b> B. Hyperactivity–Impulsivity 1. <a> <b> 2. <a> <b> 3. < > 4. <a> <b> 5. < > 6. <a> <b> 7. < > 8. <a> <b> 9. <a> <b> <c>	1. <a> <b> 2. <a> <b> 3. <a> <b> <c> <d> 4. < > 5. <a> <b> 6. < > 7. < > 8. < >	1. < > 2. <a> <b> 3. < > 4. < > 5. < > 6. < > 7. <a> <b> 8. <a> <b> 9. < > 10. <a> <b> 11. < > 12. < > 13. < > 14. < > 15. <a> <b>
Criteria If ≥6 in *A only*, then criteria met Inattentive < > If ≥6 in *B only*, then criteria met Hyperactive–Impulsive < > If ≥6 in A *and* ≥6 in B, then criteria met Combined < >	**Criteria** If ≥4, then criteria met ODD < >	**Criteria** If ≥3, then criteria met CD < >
Duration 1. ____________ (years old) 2. < > _________ (years old) 3. < > __________ (months) * DUR met for ADHD < >	**Duration** 1. ____________ (years old) 2. < > _________ (years old) 3. < > __________ (months) * DUR met for ODD < >	**Duration** 1. ____________ (years old) 2. < > _________ (years old) 3. < > __________ (months) * DUR met for CD < >
Impairment 1. < > home 2. < > school 3. < > peers	**Impairment** 1. < > home 2. < > school 3. < > peers	**Impairment** 1. < > home 2. < > school 3. < > peers **Type** Childhood Onset < > Adolescent Onset < > Mild < > Moderate < > Severe < >

SUB AB	PHO	SOCIAL PHO
1. < > <a>________________ <b>________________ <c>________________ ________________ 2. < > ________________ 3. < > ________________ 4. < > ________________	1. ________________ ________________ ________________ 2. <a> <b> 3. <a> <b> 4. <ai> <aii> <aiii> <aiv> <b> 5. <a> <b>	1. <a> <b> 2. < > 3. <a> <b> 4. <ai> <aii> <aiii> <aiv> <b> 5. < >
Duration 1. __________ (years old) 2. < > __________ (years old) __________ (months) * DUR met for SUB AB < >	**Criteria** If 1–4, then criteria met PHO < >	**Criteria** If 1–4, then criteria met SOCIAL PHO < >
	Duration 1. __________ (years old) 2. < > __________ (years old) 3. < > __________ (months) * DUR met for PHO < >	**Duration** 1. __________ (years old) 2. < > __________ (years old) 3. < > __________ (months) *DUR met for SOCIAL PHO < >
Impairment 1. <a> <b> 2. < > 3. <a> <b> 4. < >	**Impairment** 1. < > home 2. < > school 3. < > peers	**Impairment** 1. < > home 2. < > school 3. < > peers
Criteria If any use (Q1–4) and any impairment (1–4), then criteria met SUB AB < >	**Type(s)** Animal < > Natural Environment < > Blood–Injection–Injury < > Situational < > Other ____________ < >	
Type(s) ________________ ________________ ________________ ________________		

SEP ANX	GEN ANX	OCD
1. <a> <b> 2. <a> <b> 3. < > 4. <a> <b> 5. <a> <b> 6. <a> <b> 7. <a> <b> 8. <a> <b>	1. < > ______________ ______________ ______________ ______________ ______________ 2. <a> <b> 3. <a> <b> <c> <d> <e> <f>	A. Compulsions 1. < > ______________ 2. <a> ______________ <b> 3. < > B. Obsessions 1. <a> ______________ <b> ______________ <c> ______________ 2. <a> <b> <c> 3. < > C. Interference 1. <a> <b> <c>
Criteria If ≥3, then criteria met SEP ANX < >	**Criteria** If 1–3, then criteria met GEN ANX < >	**Criteria** If A1, A2, & C, then criteria met Compulsions < > If B1, B2, & C, then criteria met Obsessions < > If Compulsions + and/or Obsessions +, then criteria met OCD < >
Duration 1. ____________ (years old) 2. < > __________ (years old) 3. < > __________ (weeks) *DUR met for SEP ANX < >	**Duration** 1. ____________ (years old) 2. < > __________ (years old) 3. < > __________ (months) *DUR met for GEN ANX < >	**Duration** 1. ____________ (years old) 2. < > __________ (years old) __________ (months) *DUR met for OCD < >
Impairment 1. < > home 2. < > school 3. < > peers	**Impairment** 1. < > home 2. < > school 3. < > peers	**Impairment** 1. < > home 2. < > school 3. < > peers

STRESS (ASD/PTSD)	ANO	BUL
A. Exposure 1. <a> <b> ____________________ 2. <a> <b> <c> <d> <e> 3. < > ________________________ B. Dissociation 1. <a> <b> <c> <d> 2. < > 3. < > 4. < > 5. < > C. Reexperiencing 1. <a> <b> <c> 2. <a> <b> 3. <a> <b> 4. <a> <b> 5. < > D. Avoidance 1. <a> <b> 2. <a> <b> <c> 3. < > 4. <a> <b> 5. <a> <b> 6. <a> <b> 7. <a> <b> E. Hyperarousal 1. <a> <b> 2. <a> <b> 3. < > 4. < > 5. < >	1. <a> <b> 2. <a> ht: ______________ wt: ______________ <b> ht: ______________ wt: ______________ 3. <a> <b> <c> 4. <a> <b> <c> 5. < >	1. < > ____________________ ____________________ 2. <a> <b> <c> <d> 3. <a> <b> <c> <d> 4. <a> <b>
Criteria If A1 & A2, ≥3 in B, ≥1 in C, ≥3 in D, and ≥2 in E, then criteria met ASD < > If A1 & A2, ≥1 in C, ≥3 in D, and ≥2 in E, then criteria met PTSD < >	**Criteria** If 1–4 (&5 for pubescent girls), then criteria met ANO < >	**Criteria** If 1–4, then criteria met BUL < >
Duration 1. ______________ (years old) 2. < > __________ (years old) 3. a. < > _______ (weeks) b. < > c. < > _______ (days) 4. < > ___________ (months) *DUR met for ASD < > *DUR met for PTSD < >	**Duration** 1. ___________ (years old) 2. < > ________ (years old) 3. < > ________ (months) *DUR met for ANO < >	**Duration** 1. ___________ (years old) 2. < > ________ (years old) 3. a. < > _____ (#/week) b. < > _____ (months) *DUR met for BUL < >
Impairment 1. < > home 2. < > school 3. < > peers **Type (PTSD)** Acute < > Regular Onset < > Chronic < > Delayed Onset < >	**Impairment** 1. < > home 2. < > school 3. < > peers	**Impairment** 1. < > home 2. < > school 3. < > peers

DEP/DYS (MDD/DD)

A. Dysphoric Mood
  1. <a> <b> <c>
  2. <a> <bi> <bii> <biii>
     <c> <d>

B. Loss of Interest
  1. <a> <b>
  2. <a> <b> <c>

C. Appetite Changes
  1. <a> <b> <c>
  2. <a> <b>

D. Sleep Changes
  Bedtime: __________
  Wakeup: __________
  1. <a> <b> <c>
  2. <a> <b>

E. Psychomotor Changes
  1. <a> <b> <c> <d>
  2. <a> <b>

F. Low Energy
  1. <a> <b> <c> <d>

G. Guilt
  1. <a> <b> <c> <d>
  2. <a> <b>

H. Impaired Concentration
  1. <a> <b> <c> <d> <e>
  2. < >

I. Hopelessness
  1. <a> <b> <c>

J. Morbid/Suicidal Thoughts
  1. <a> <b>
  2. <a> <b> <c> <d> <e>

____
____
____
____
____

DEP/DYS (MDD/DD)

Criteria

If A &/or B & ≥5 of A–H or J,
then criteria met
MDD < >

If A & ≥2 of C, D, F, G, H, or I,
then criteria met
DD < >

Duration

1. ______________ (years old)
2. < > ____________ (years old)
3. MDD < > ________ (weeks)
   DD < > _________ (months)

*DUR met for MDD < >
*DUR met for DD < >

Impairment

1. < > home
2. < > school
3. < > peers

MAN/HYPOMAN

A. Elevated Mood
  1. <a> ____________________
     <b> ____________________
     <c> ____________________
  2. < > ____________________

B. Other Symptoms
  1. <a> ____________________
     <b>
  2. <a> <b> <c> ____________
  3. <a> <b> <c> <d>
  4. <a> <b> <c>
  5. < >
  6. <a> <b> <c> <d> <e>
  7. <a> <b> <c> <d>

C. Interference
  1. < >
  2. < >

Criteria

If A1(a, b, & c) + ≥3 in B + ≥1 in C
or
A2 + ≥4 in B + ≥1 in C,
then criteria met
MAN < >

If A1(a, b, & c) + ≥3 in B +
none in C
or
A2 + ≥4 in B + none in C,
then criteria met
HYPOMAN < >

Duration

1. ______________ (years old)
2. < > ____________ (years old)
3. MAN < > ________ (weeks)
   HYPO < > _______ (days)

*DUR met for MAN < >
*DUR met for HYPOMAN < >

Impairment

1. < > home
2. < > school
3. < > peers

ENU

1. < >
2. <a> <b>
3. <a> <b>

Criteria

If 1, ≥1 in 2, 3a, and 3b, then criteria met

ENU < >

Duration

1. ____________ (years old)
2. < > __________ (years old)
3. <a> __________ (x/week)
   <b> __________ (months)

*DUR met for ENU < >

Impairment

1. < > home
2. < > school
3. < > peers

Type

Nocturnal	< >
Diurnal	< >
Both	< >

ENC

1. < >
2. < >

Criteria

If both 1 & 2, then criteria met

ENC < >

Duration

1. ____________ (years old)
2. < > __________ (years old)
3. <a> __________ (x/month)
   <b> __________ (months)

*DUR met for ENC < >

Impairment

1. < > home
2. < > school
3. < > peers

SCZ/PSY

A. Psychotic Symptoms
1. <a> <b> <c> <d> <e>
2. <a> <b> <c> <d> <e> <f>
3. < >
4. < >
5. < >

B. Interference
1. < >
2. < >
3. < >

Criteria

If ≥2 in A and ≥1 in B, then criteria met

SCZ < >

If ≥1 in A, then criteria met

PSY < >

Duration

1. ______________ (years old)
2. < > ___________ (years old)
3. < > ___________ (months)

*DUR met for SCZ < >

*DUR met for PSY < >

Impairment

1. < > home
2. < > school
3. < > peers

STRESSORS

A. Child Abuse/Neglect
1. <a> <b> <c>
2. <a> <b> <c> <d>
3. <a> <b> <c> <d>
4. < >
5. < >

Duration

1. ______________________
2. < > __________________
3. ______________________
4. ______________________
5. < >

B. Other Stressors
1. <a> <b> <c> <d> <e>
2. < >
3. <a> <b>
4. <a> <b> <c>
5. <a> <b>
6. <a> <b>
7. <a> ______________
   <b>
8. <a> <b> <c> <d>
9. < > ______________
   ____
   ____
10. < >
11. < > ______________
   ____
   ____

P-ChIPS Scoring Form
Profile Sheet

Child's Number: ______________________ Date: ______________

Child's Name: ______________________ Time Started: ______________

Date of Birth: ______________ Age: ______________ Time Ended: ______________

Race: ______________ Sex: ______________ Interviewer: ______________

Informant's Name: ______________________

Informant's Relationship (circle one): Mother, Father, Stepmother, Stepfather, Guardian, Other: ______________

	Disorder	Symptoms	Diagnosis	Duration	Clinician's Diagnosis
ADHD	**Attention-Deficit/Hyperactivity Disorder** *Type:* Inattentive, Hyperactive–Impulsive, Combined	<>	<>	<>	**Axis I**
ODD	**Oppositional Defiant Disorder**	<>	<>	<>	
CD	**Conduct Disorder** *Onset:* Childhood, Adolescent *Severity:* Mild, Moderate, Severe	<>	<>	<>	
SUBAB	**Substance Abuse** *Substance(s):* ______________	<>	<>	<>	
PHO	**Specific Phobia** *Type:* ______________	<>	<>	<>	**Axis II**
SOCPHO	**Social Phobia**	<>	<>	<>	
SEPANX	**Separation Anxiety Disorder**	<>	<>	<>	**Axis III**
GENANX	**General Anxiety Disorder**	<>	<>	<>	
OCD	**Obsessive-Compulsive Disorder**	<>	<>	<>	
PTSD	**Posttraumatic Stress Disorder** *Type:* Acute, Chronic *Onset:* Regular, Delayed	<>	<>	<>	**Axis IV**
ASD	**Acute Stress Disorder**	<>	<>	<>	
ANO	**Anorexia**	<>	<>	<>	**Axis V**
BUL	**Bulimia**	<>	<>	<>	**current:**
DEP	**Major Depressive Disorder**	<>	<>	<>	**past year:**
DYS	**Dysthymic Disorder**	<>	<>	<>	
MAN	**Mania**	<>	<>	<>	
HYPOMAN	**Hypomania**	<>	<>	<>	
ENU	**Enuresis** *Type:* Nocturnal, Diurnal, Both	<>	<>	<>	
ENC	**Encopresis**	<>	<>	<>	
SCZ	**Schizophrenia**	<>	<>	<>	
PSY	**Psychosis**	<>	<>	<>	

Psychosocial Stressors:

Other Stressors:

Behavioral Observations

Appearance:

Affect:

Effort:

Level of Activity:

Unusual Behaviors:

Presenting Problem

Home

1.

2.

School

1.

2.

3.

4.

5.

Peers/Work

1.

2.

3.

4.

5.

Medication

Type:

Dosage:

Child's Name: ____________________

Date: ____________

ADHD	ODD	CD
A. Inattention 1. <a> <b> 2. < > 3. <a> <b> 4. <a> <b> <c> 5. < > 6. < > 7. < > 8. <a> <b> 9. <a> <b> B. Hyperactivity–Impulsivity 1. <a> <b> 2. <a> <b> 3. < > 4. <a> <b> 5. < > 6. <a> <b> 7. < > 8. <a> <b> 9. <a> <b> <c>	1. <a> <b> 2. <a> <b> 3. <a> <b> <c> <d> 4. < > 5. <a> <b> 6. < > 7. < > 8. < >	1. < > 2. <a> <b> 3. < > 4. < > 5. < > 6. < > 7. <a> <b> 8. <a> <b> 9. < > 10. <a> <b> 11. < > 12. < > 13. < > 14. < > 15. <a> <b>
Criteria If ≥6 in *A only*, then criteria met Inattentive < > If ≥6 in *B only*, then criteria met Hyperactive–Impulsive < > If ≥6 in A *and* ≥6 in B, then criteria met Combined < >	**Criteria** If ≥4, then criteria met ODD < >	**Criteria** If ≥3, then criteria met CD < >
Duration 1. __________ (years old) 2. < > ________ (years old) 3. < > ________ (months) * DUR met for ADHD < >	**Duration** 1. __________ (years old) 2. < > ________ (years old) 3. < > ________ (months) * DUR met for ODD < >	**Duration** 1. __________ (years old) 2. < > ________ (years old) 3. < > ________ (months) * DUR met for CD < >
Impairment 1. < > home 2. < > school 3. < > peers	**Impairment** 1. < > home 2. < > school 3. < > peers	**Impairment** 1. < > home 2. < > school 3. < > peers
		Type Childhood Onset < > Adolescent Onset < > Mild < > Moderate < > Severe < >

SUB AB

1. < >
   <a>________________
   <b>________________
   <c>________________
   ____
2. < > ________________
3. < > ________________
4. < > ________________

Duration

1. ____________ (years old)
2. < > __________ (years old)
   __________ (months)

* DUR met for SUB AB < >

Impairment

1. <a> <b>
2. < >
3. <a> <b>
4. < >

Criteria

If any use (Q1–4) and any impairment (1–4), then criteria met SUB AB < >

Type(s) ________________
____
____
____

PHO

1. ________________
   ____
   ____
2. <a> <b>
3. <a> <b>
4. <ai> <aii> <aiii> <aiv> <b>
5. <a> <b>

Criteria

If 1–4, then criteria met PHO < >

Duration

1. ____________ (years old)
2. < > __________ (years old)
3. < > __________ (months)

* DUR met for PHO < >

Impairment

1. < > home
2. < > school
3. < > peers

Type(s)

Animal	< >
Natural Environment	< >
Blood–Injection–Injury	< >
Situational	< >
Other ________________	< >

SOCIAL PHO

1. <a> <b>
2. < >
3. <a> <b>
4. <ai> <aii> <aiii> <aiv> <b>
5. < >

Criteria

If 1–4, then criteria met SOCIAL PHO < >

Duration

1. ____________ (years old)
2. < > __________ (years old)
3. < > __________ (months)

*DUR met for SOCIAL PHO < >

Impairment

1. < > home
2. < > school
3. < > peers

SEP ANX	GEN ANX	OCD
1. <a> <b> 2. <a> <b> 3. < > 4. <a> <b> 5. <a> <b> 6. <a> <b> 7. <a> <b> 8. <a> <b>	1. < > ____________ ____________ ____________ ____________ ____________ 2. <a> <b> 3. <a> <b> <c> <d> <e> <f>	A. Compulsions 1. < > ____________ 2. <a> ____________ <b> 3. < > B. Obsessions 1. <a> ____________ <b> ____________ <c> ____________ 2. <a> <b> <c> 3. < > C. Interference 1. <a> <b> <c>
Criteria If ≥3, then criteria met SEP ANX < >	**Criteria** If 1–3, then criteria met GEN ANX < >	**Criteria** If A1, A2, & C, then criteria met Compulsions < > If B1, B2, & C, then criteria met Obsessions < > If Compulsions + and/or Obsessions +, then criteria met OCD < >
Duration 1. ____________ (years old) 2. < > ________ (years old) 3. < > ________ (weeks) *DUR met for SEP ANX < >	**Duration** 1. ____________ (years old) 2. < > ________ (years old) 3. < > ________ (months) *DUR met for GEN ANX < >	**Duration** 1. ____________ (years old) 2. < > ________ (years old) ________ (months) *DUR met for OCD < >
Impairment 1. < > home 2. < > school 3. < > peers	**Impairment** 1. < > home 2. < > school 3. < > peers	**Impairment** 1. < > home 2. < > school 3. < > peers

STRESS (ASD/PTSD)	ANO	BUL
A. Exposure 1. <a> <b> ______________ 2. <a> <b> <c> <d> <e> 3. < > __________________ B. Dissociation 1. <a> <b> <c> <d> 2. < > 3. < > 4. < > 5. < > C. Reexperiencing 1. <a> <b> <c> 2. <a> <b> 3. <a> <b> 4. <a> <b> 5. < > D. Avoidance 1. <a> <b> 2. <a> <b> <c> 3. < > 4. <a> <b> 5. <a> <b> 6. <a> <b> 7. <a> <b> E. Hyperarousal 1. <a> <b> 2. <a> <b> 3. < > 4. < > 5. < >	1. <a> <b> 2. <a> ht: ____________ wt: ____________ <b> ht: ____________ wt: ____________ 3. <a> <b> <c> 4. <a> <b> <c> 5. < >	1. < > ______________ ______________________ 2. <a> <b> <c> <d> 3. <a> <b> <c> <d> 4. <a> <b>
Criteria If A1 & A2, ≥3 in B, ≥1 in C, ≥3 in D, and ≥2 in E, then criteria met ASD < > If A1 & A2, ≥1 in C, ≥3 in D, and ≥2 in E, then criteria met PTSD < >	**Criteria** If 1–4 (&5 for pubescent girls), then criteria met ANO < >	**Criteria** If 1–4, then criteria met BUL < >
Duration 1. ____________ (years old) 2. < > __________ (years old) 3. a. < > _______ (weeks) b. < > c. < > _______ (days) 4. < > __________ (months) *DUR met for ASD < > *DUR met for PTSD < >	**Duration** 1. _________ (years old) 2. < > _______ (years old) 3. < > _______ (months) *DUR met for ANO < >	**Duration** 1. _________ (years old) 2. < > _______ (years old) 3. a. < > _____ (#/week) b. < > _____ (months) *DUR met for BUL < >
Impairment 1. < > home 2. < > school 3. < > peers **Type (PTSD)** Acute < > Regular Onset < > Chronic < > Delayed Onset < >	**Impairment** 1. < > home 2. < > school 3. < > peers	**Impairment** 1. < > home 2. < > school 3. < > peers

DEP/DYS (MDD/DD)

A. Dysphoric Mood
1. <a> <b> <c>
2. <a> <bi> <bii> <biii> <c> <d>

B. Loss of Interest
1. <a> <b>
2. <a> <b> <c>

C. Appetite Changes
1. <a> <b> <c>
2. <a> <b>

D. Sleep Changes
Bedtime: __________
Wakeup: __________
1. <a> <b> <c>
2. <a> <b>

E. Psychomotor Changes
1. <a> <b> <c> <d>
2. <a> <b>

F. Low Energy
1. <a> <b> <c> <d>

G. Guilt
1. <a> <b> <c> <d>
2. <a> <b>

H. Impaired Concentration
1. <a> <b> <c> <d> <e>
2. < >

I. Hopelessness
1. <a> <b> <c>

J. Morbid/Suicidal Thoughts
1. <a> <b>
2. <a> <b> <c> <d> <e>

____
____
____
____
____

DEP/DYS (MDD/DD)

Criteria

If A &/or B & ≥5 of A–H or J, then criteria met MDD < >

If A & ≥2 of C, D, F, G, H, or I, then criteria met DD < >

Duration
1. ______________ (years old)
2. < > ____________ (years old)
3. MDD < > ________ (weeks)
   DD < > ________ (months)

*DUR met for MDD < >
*DUR met for DD < >

Impairment
1. < > home
2. < > school
3. < > peers

MAN/HYPOMAN

A. Elevated Mood
1. <a> ______________________
   <b> ______________________
   <c> ______________________
2. < > ______________________

B. Other Symptoms
1. <a> ______________________
   <b>
2. <a> <b> <c> ____________
3. <a> <b> <c> <d>
4. <a> <b> <c>
5. < >
6. <a> <b> <c> <d> <e>
7. <a> <b> <c> <d>

C. Interference
1. < >
2. < >

Criteria

If A1(a, b, & c) + ≥3 in B + ≥1 in C
or
A2 + ≥4 in B + ≥1 in C,
then criteria met
MAN < >

If A1(a, b, & c) + ≥3 in B + none in C
or
A2 + ≥4 in B + none in C,
then criteria met
HYPOMAN < >

Duration
1. ______________ (years old)
2. < > ____________ (years old)
3. MAN < > ________ (weeks)
   HYPO < > ________ (days)

*DUR met for MAN < >
*DUR met for HYPOMAN < >

Impairment
1. < > home
2. < > school
3. < > peers

ENU

1. < >
2. <a> <b>
3. <a> <b>

Criteria

If 1, ≥1 in 2, 3a, and 3b, then criteria met
ENU < >

Duration

1. ____________ (years old)
2. < > ________ (years old)
3. <a> ________ (x/week)
   <b> ________ (months)

*DUR met for ENU < >

Impairment

1. < > home
2. < > school
3. < > peers

Type

Nocturnal	< >
Diurnal	< >
Both	< >

ENC

1. < >
2. < >

Criteria

If both 1 & 2, then criteria met
ENC < >

Duration

1. ____________ (years old)
2. < > ________ (years old)
3. <a> ________ (x/month)
   <b> ________ (months)

*DUR met for ENC < >

Impairment

1. < > home
2. < > school
3. < > peers

SCZ/PSY

A. Psychotic Symptoms
   1. <a> <b> <c> <d> <e>
   2. <a> <b> <c> <d> <e> <f>
   3. < >
   4. < >
   5. < >

B. Interference
   1. < >
   2. < >
   3. < >

Criteria

If ≥2 in A and ≥1 in B, then criteria met
SCZ < >

If ≥1 in A, then criteria met
PSY < >

Duration

1. ______________ (years old)
2. < > ___________ (years old)
3. < > ___________ (months)

*DUR met for SCZ < >
*DUR met for PSY < >

Impairment

1. < > home
2. < > school
3. < > peers

STRESSORS

A. Child Abuse/Neglect
   1. <a> <b> <c>
   2. <a> <b> <c> <d>
   3. <a> <b> <c> <d>
   4. < >
   5. < >

Duration

1. ______________________
2. < > __________________
3. ______________________
4. ______________________
5. < >

B. Other Stressors
   1. <a> <b> <c> <d> <e>
   2. < >
   3. <a> <b>
   4. <a> <b> <c>
   5. <a> <b>
   6. <a> <b>
   7. <a> ______________
      <b>
   8. <a> <b> <c> <d>
   9. < > ______________
      ____
      ____
   10. < >
   11. < > ______________
      ____
      ____

P-ChIPS Scoring Form
Profile Sheet

Child's Number: ____________________ Date: ____________

Child's Name: ____________________ Time Started: ____________

Date of Birth: ____________ Age: ____________ Time Ended: ____________

Race: ____________ Sex: ____________ Interviewer: ____________

Informant's Name: ____________________

Informant's Relationship (circle one): Mother, Father, Stepmother, Stepfather, Guardian, Other: ____________

	Disorder	Symptoms	Diagnosis	Duration	Clinician's Diagnosis
ADHD	**Attention-Deficit/Hyperactivity Disorder**	<>	<>	<>	**Axis I**
	Type: Inattentive, Hyperactive–Impulsive, Combined				
ODD	**Oppositional Defiant Disorder**	<>	<>	<>	
CD	**Conduct Disorder**	<>	<>	<>	
	Onset: Childhood, Adolescent				
	Severity: Mild, Moderate, Severe				
SUBAB	**Substance Abuse**	<>	<>	<>	
	Substance(s): ____________				
PHO	**Specific Phobia**	<>	<>	<>	**Axis II**
	Type: ____________				
SOCPHO	**Social Phobia**	<>	<>	<>	
SEPANX	**Separation Anxiety Disorder**	<>	<>	<>	**Axis III**
GENANX	**General Anxiety Disorder**	<>	<>	<>	
OCD	**Obsessive-Compulsive Disorder**	<>	<>	<>	
PTSD	**Posttraumatic Stress Disorder**	<>	<>	<>	**Axis IV**
	Type: Acute, Chronic				
	Onset: Regular, Delayed				
ASD	**Acute Stress Disorder**	<>	<>	<>	
ANO	**Anorexia**	<>	<>	<>	**Axis V**
BUL	**Bulimia**	<>	<>	<>	**current:**
DEP	**Major Depressive Disorder**	<>	<>	<>	**past year:**
DYS	**Dysthymic Disorder**	<>	<>	<>	
MAN	**Mania**	<>	<>	<>	
HYPOMAN	**Hypomania**	<>	<>	<>	
ENU	**Enuresis**	<>	<>	<>	
	Type: Nocturnal, Diurnal, Both				
ENC	**Encopresis**	<>	<>	<>	
SCZ	**Schizophrenia**	<>	<>	<>	
PSY	**Psychosis**	<>	<>	<>	

Psychosocial Stressors:

Other Stressors:

Behavioral Observations

Appearance:

Affect:

Effort:

Level of Activity:

Unusual Behaviors:

Presenting Problem

Home

1.

2.

School

1.

2.

3.

4.

5.

Peers/Work

1.

2.

3.

4.

5.

Medication

Type:

Dosage:

Child's Name: ______________________________

Date: _______________

ADHD	ODD	CD
A. Inattention 1. <a> <b> 2. < > 3. <a> <b> 4. <a> <b> <c> 5. < > 6. < > 7. < > 8. <a> <b> 9. <a> <b> B. Hyperactivity–Impulsivity 1. <a> <b> 2. <a> <b> 3. < > 4. <a> <b> 5. < > 6. <a> <b> 7. < > 8. <a> <b> 9. <a> <b> <c>	1. <a> <b> 2. <a> <b> 3. <a> <b> <c> <d> 4. < > 5. <a> <b> 6. < > 7. < > 8. < >	1. < > 2. <a> <b> 3. < > 4. < > 5. < > 6. < > 7. <a> <b> 8. <a> <b> 9. < > 10. <a> <b> 11. < > 12. < > 13. < > 14. < > 15. <a> <b>
Criteria If ≥6 in *A only*, then criteria met Inattentive < > If ≥6 in *B only*, then criteria met Hyperactive–Impulsive < > If ≥6 in A *and* ≥6 in B, then criteria met Combined < >	**Criteria** If ≥4, then criteria met ODD < >	**Criteria** If ≥3, then criteria met CD < >
Duration 1. ___________ (years old) 2. < > _________ (years old) 3. < > _________ (months) * DUR met for ADHD < >	**Duration** 1. ___________ (years old) 2. < > _________ (years old) 3. < > _________ (months) * DUR met for ODD < >	**Duration** 1. ___________ (years old) 2. < > _________ (years old) 3. < > _________ (months) * DUR met for CD < >
Impairment 1. < > home 2. < > school 3. < > peers	**Impairment** 1. < > home 2. < > school 3. < > peers	**Impairment** 1. < > home 2. < > school 3. < > peers **Type** Childhood Onset < > Adolescent Onset < > Mild < > Moderate < > Severe < >

SUB AB

1. < >
   <a>____________________
   <b>____________________
   <c>____________________
   ____
2. < > ____________________
3. < > ____________________
4. < > ____________________

Duration

1. ____________ (years old)
2. < > __________ (years old)
   __________ (months)

* DUR met for SUB AB < >

Impairment

1. <a> <b>
2. < >
3. <a> <b>
4. < >

Criteria

If any use (Q1–4) and any impairment (1–4), then criteria met SUB AB < >

Type(s) ____________________
____
____
____

PHO

1. ____________________
   ____
   ____
2. <a> <b>
3. <a> <b>
4. <ai> <aii> <aiii> <aiv> <b>
5. <a> <b>

Criteria

If 1–4, then criteria met
PHO < >

Duration

1. ____________ (years old)
2. < > __________ (years old)
3. < > __________ (months)

* DUR met for PHO < >

Impairment

1. < > home
2. < > school
3. < > peers

Type(s)

Animal	< >
Natural Environment	< >
Blood–Injection–Injury	< >
Situational	< >
Other ________________	< >

SOCIAL PHO

1. <a> <b>
2. < >
3. <a> <b>
4. <ai> <aii> <aiii> <aiv> <b>
5. < >

Criteria

If 1–4, then criteria met
SOCIAL PHO < >

Duration

1. ____________ (years old)
2. < > __________ (years old)
3. < > __________ (months)

*DUR met for SOCIAL PHO < >

Impairment

1. < > home
2. < > school
3. < > peers

SEP ANX	GEN ANX	OCD
1. <a> <b> 2. <a> <b> 3. < > 4. <a> <b> 5. <a> <b> 6. <a> <b> 7. <a> <b> 8. <a> <b>	1. < > ____________ ____________ ____________ ____________ ____________ 2. <a> <b> 3. <a> <b> <c> <d> <e> <f>	A. Compulsions 1. < > ____________ 2. <a> ____________ <b> 3. < > B. Obsessions 1. <a> ____________ <b> ____________ <c> ____________ 2. <a> <b> <c> 3. < > C. Interference 1. <a> <b> <c>
Criteria If ≥3, then criteria met SEP ANX < >	**Criteria** If 1–3, then criteria met GEN ANX < >	**Criteria** If A1, A2, & C, then criteria met Compulsions < > If B1, B2, & C, then criteria met Obsessions < > If Compulsions + and/or Obsessions +, then criteria met OCD < >
Duration 1. ____________ (years old) 2. < > __________ (years old) 3. < > __________ (weeks) *DUR met for SEP ANX < >	**Duration** 1. ____________ (years old) 2. < > __________ (years old) 3. < > __________ (months) *DUR met for GEN ANX < >	**Duration** 1. ____________ (years old) 2. < > __________ (years old) __________ (months) *DUR met for OCD < >
Impairment 1. < > home 2. < > school 3. < > peers	**Impairment** 1. < > home 2. < > school 3. < > peers	**Impairment** 1. < > home 2. < > school 3. < > peers

STRESS (ASD/PTSD)	ANO	BUL
A. Exposure 1. <a> <b> ________________ 2. <a> <b> <c> <d> <e> 3. < > ____________________ B. Dissociation 1. <a> <b> <c> <d> 2. < > 3. < > 4. < > 5. < > C. Reexperiencing 1. <a> <b> <c> 2. <a> <b> 3. <a> <b> 4. <a> <b> 5. < > D. Avoidance 1. <a> <b> 2. <a> <b> <c> 3. < > 4. <a> <b> 5. <a> <b> 6. <a> <b> 7. <a> <b> E. Hyperarousal 1. <a> <b> 2. <a> <b> 3. < > 4. < > 5. < >	1. <a> <b> 2. <a> ht: ____________ wt: ____________ <b> ht: ____________ wt: ____________ 3. <a> <b> <c> 4. <a> <b> <c> 5. < >	1. < > ________________ ________________________ 2. <a> <b> <c> <d> 3. <a> <b> <c> <d> 4. <a> <b>
Criteria If A1 & A2, ≥3 in B, ≥1 in C, ≥3 in D, and ≥2 in E, then criteria met ASD < > If A1 & A2, ≥1 in C, ≥3 in D, and ≥2 in E, then criteria met PTSD < >	**Criteria** If 1–4 (&5 for pubescent girls), then criteria met ANO < >	**Criteria** If 1–4, then criteria met BUL < >
Duration 1. ____________ (years old) 2. < > __________ (years old) 3. a. < > _______ (weeks) b. < > c. < > _______ (days) 4. < > __________ (months) *DUR met for ASD < > *DUR met for PTSD < >	**Duration** 1. __________ (years old) 2. < > _______ (years old) 3. < > _______ (months) *DUR met for ANO < >	**Duration** 1. __________ (years old) 2. < > _______ (years old) 3. a. < > _____ (#/week) b. < > _____ (months) *DUR met for BUL < >
Impairment 1. < > home 2. < > school 3. < > peers **Type (PTSD)** Acute < > Regular Onset < > Chronic < > Delayed Onset < >	**Impairment** 1. < > home 2. < > school 3. < > peers	**Impairment** 1. < > home 2. < > school 3. < > peers

DEP/DYS (MDD/DD)

A. Dysphoric Mood
1. <a> <b> <c>
2. <a> <bi> <bii> <biii> <c> <d>

B. Loss of Interest
1. <a> <b>
2. <a> <b> <c>

C. Appetite Changes
1. <a> <b> <c>
2. <a> <b>

D. Sleep Changes
Bedtime: __________
Wakeup: __________
1. <a> <b> <c>
2. <a> <b>

E. Psychomotor Changes
1. <a> <b> <c> <d>
2. <a> <b>

F. Low Energy
1. <a> <b> <c> <d>

G. Guilt
1. <a> <b> <c> <d>
2. <a> <b>

H. Impaired Concentration
1. <a> <b> <c> <d> <e>
2. < >

I. Hopelessness
1. <a> <b> <c>

J. Morbid/Suicidal Thoughts
1. <a> <b>
2. <a> <b> <c> <d> <e>

____
____
____
____
____

DEP/DYS (MDD/DD)

Criteria

If A &/or B & ≥5 of A–H or J, then criteria met MDD < >

If A & ≥2 of C, D, F, G, H, or I, then criteria met DD < >

Duration

1. ______________ (years old)
2. < > ___________ (years old)
3. MDD < > _______ (weeks)
   DD < > ________ (months)

*DUR met for MDD < >
*DUR met for DD < >

Impairment

1. < > home
2. < > school
3. < > peers

MAN/HYPOMAN

A. Elevated Mood
1. <a> ____________________
   <b> ____________________
   <c> ____________________
2. < > ____________________

B. Other Symptoms
1. <a> ____________________
   <b>
2. <a> <b> <c> ___________
3. <a> <b> <c> <d>
4. <a> <b> <c>
5. < >
6. <a> <b> <c> <d> <e>
7. <a> <b> <c> <d>

C. Interference
1. < >
2. < >

Criteria

If A1(a, b, & c) + ≥3 in B + ≥1 in C *or* A2 + ≥4 in B + ≥1 in C, then criteria met MAN < >

If A1(a, b, & c) + ≥3 in B + none in C *or* A2 + ≥4 in B + none in C, then criteria met HYPOMAN < >

Duration

1. ______________ (years old)
2. < > ___________ (years old)
3. MAN < > _______ (weeks)
   HYPO < > ______ (days)

*DUR met for MAN < >
*DUR met for HYPOMAN < >

Impairment

1. < > home
2. < > school
3. < > peers

ENU

1. < >
2. <a> <b>
3. <a> <b>

Criteria

If 1, ≥1 in 2, 3a, and 3b, then criteria met
ENU < >

Duration

1. __________ (years old)
2. < > __________ (years old)
3. <a> __________ (x/week)
   <b> __________ (months)

*DUR met for ENU < >

Impairment

1. < > home
2. < > school
3. < > peers

Type

Nocturnal < >
Diurnal < >
Both < >

ENC

1. < >
2. < >

Criteria

If both 1 & 2, then criteria met
ENC < >

Duration

1. __________ (years old)
2. < > __________ (years old)
3. <a> __________ (x/month)
   <b> __________ (months)

*DUR met for ENC < >

Impairment

1. < > home
2. < > school
3. < > peers

SCZ/PSY

A. Psychotic Symptoms
1. <a> <b> <c> <d> <e>
2. <a> <b> <c> <d> <e> <f>
3. < >
4. < >
5. < >

B. Interference
1. < >
2. < >
3. < >

Criteria

If ≥2 in A and ≥1 in B, then criteria met
SCZ < >

If ≥1 in A, then criteria met
PSY < >

Duration

1. __________ (years old)
2. < > __________ (years old)
3. < > __________ (months)

*DUR met for SCZ < >
*DUR met for PSY < >

Impairment

1. < > home
2. < > school
3. < > peers

STRESSORS

A. Child Abuse/Neglect
1. <a> <b> <c>
2. <a> <b> <c> <d>
3. <a> <b> <c> <d>
4. < >
5. < >

Duration

1. __________
2. < > __________
3. __________
4. __________
5. < >

B. Other Stressors
1. <a> <b> <c> <d> <e>
2. < >
3. <a> <b>
4. <a> <b> <c>
5. <a> <b>
6. <a> <b>
7. <a> __________
   <b>
8. <a> <b> <c> <d>
9. < > __________
   ____
   ____
10. < >
11. < > __________
   ____
   ____

P-ChIPS Scoring Form
Profile Sheet

Child's Number: ______________________ Date: ______________

Child's Name: ______________________ Time Started: ______________

Date of Birth: ______________ Age: ______________ Time Ended: ______________

Race: ______________ Sex: ______________ Interviewer: ______________

Informant's Name: ______________________

Informant's Relationship (circle one): Mother, Father, Stepmother, Stepfather, Guardian, Other: ______________

	Disorder	Symptoms	Diagnosis	Duration	Clinician's Diagnosis
ADHD	**Attention-Deficit/Hyperactivity Disorder**	<>	<>	<>	**Axis I**
	Type: Inattentive, Hyperactive–Impulsive, Combined				
ODD	**Oppositional Defiant Disorder**	<>	<>	<>	
CD	**Conduct Disorder**	<>	<>	<>	
	Onset: Childhood, Adolescent				
	Severity: Mild, Moderate, Severe				
SUBAB	**Substance Abuse**	<>	<>	<>	
	Substance(s): ______________				
PHO	**Specific Phobia**	<>	<>	<>	**Axis II**
	Type: ______________				
SOCPHO	**Social Phobia**	<>	<>	<>	
SEPANX	**Separation Anxiety Disorder**	<>	<>	<>	**Axis III**
GENANX	**General Anxiety Disorder**	<>	<>	<>	
OCD	**Obsessive-Compulsive Disorder**	<>	<>	<>	
PTSD	**Posttraumatic Stress Disorder**	<>	<>	<>	**Axis IV**
	Type: Acute, Chronic				
	Onset: Regular, Delayed				
ASD	**Acute Stress Disorder**	<>	<>	<>	
ANO	**Anorexia**	<>	<>	<>	**Axis V**
BUL	**Bulimia**	<>	<>	<>	**current:**
DEP	**Major Depressive Disorder**	<>	<>	<>	**past year:**
DYS	**Dysthymic Disorder**	<>	<>	<>	
MAN	**Mania**	<>	<>	<>	
HYPOMAN	**Hypomania**	<>	<>	<>	
ENU	**Enuresis**	<>	<>	<>	
	Type: Nocturnal, Diurnal, Both				
ENC	**Encopresis**	<>	<>	<>	
SCZ	**Schizophrenia**	<>	<>	<>	
PSY	**Psychosis**	<>	<>	<>	

Psychosocial Stressors:

Other Stressors:

Behavioral Observations

Appearance:

Affect:

Effort:

Level of Activity:

Unusual Behaviors:

Presenting Problem

Home

1.

2.

School

1.

2.

3.

4.

5.

Peers/Work

1.

2.

3.

4.

5.

Medication

Type:

Dosage:

Child's Name: ______________________________

Date: ______________

ADHD	ODD	CD
A. Inattention 1. <a> <b> 2. < > 3. <a> <b> 4. <a> <b> <c> 5. < > 6. < > 7. < > 8. <a> <b> 9. <a> <b> B. Hyperactivity–Impulsivity 1. <a> <b> 2. <a> <b> 3. < > 4. <a> <b> 5. < > 6. <a> <b> 7. < > 8. <a> <b> 9. <a> <b> <c>	1. <a> <b> 2. <a> <b> 3. <a> <b> <c> <d> 4. < > 5. <a> <b> 6. < > 7. < > 8. < >	1. < > 2. <a> <b> 3. < > 4. < > 5. < > 6. < > 7. <a> <b> 8. <a> <b> 9. < > 10. <a> <b> 11. < > 12. < > 13. < > 14. < > 15. <a> <b>
Criteria If ≥6 in *A only*, then criteria met Inattentive < > If ≥6 in *B only*, then criteria met Hyperactive–Impulsive < > If ≥6 in A *and* ≥6 in B, then criteria met Combined < >	**Criteria** If ≥4, then criteria met ODD < >	**Criteria** If ≥3, then criteria met CD < >
Duration 1. ____________ (years old) 2. < > _________ (years old) 3. < > __________ (months) * DUR met for ADHD < >	**Duration** 1. ____________ (years old) 2. < > _________ (years old) 3. < > __________ (months) * DUR met for ODD < >	**Duration** 1. ____________ (years old) 2. < > _________ (years old) 3. < > __________ (months) * DUR met for CD < >
Impairment 1. < > home 2. < > school 3. < > peers	**Impairment** 1. < > home 2. < > school 3. < > peers	**Impairment** 1. < > home 2. < > school 3. < > peers **Type** Childhood Onset < > Adolescent Onset < > Mild < > Moderate < > Severe < >

SUB AB

1. < >
   <a>______________________
   <b>______________________
   <c>______________________
   ____
2. < > ______________________
3. < > ______________________
4. < > ______________________

Duration
1. ____________ (years old)
2. < > __________ (years old)
   __________ (months)

* DUR met for SUB AB < >

Impairment
1. <a> <b>
2. < >
3. <a> <b>
4. < >

Criteria
If any use (Q1–4) and any impairment (1–4), then criteria met SUB AB < >

Type(s) ______________________
____
____
____

PHO

1. ______________________
   ____
   ____
2. <a> <b>
3. <a> <b>
4. <ai> <aii> <aiii> <aiv> <b>
5. <a> <b>

Criteria
If 1–4, then criteria met PHO < >

Duration
1. ____________ (years old)
2. < > __________ (years old)
3. < > __________ (months)

* DUR met for PHO < >

Impairment
1. < > home
2. < > school
3. < > peers

Type(s)

Animal	< >
Natural Environment	< >
Blood–Injection–Injury	< >
Situational	< >
Other ______________	< >

SOCIAL PHO

1. <a> <b>
2. < >
3. <a> <b>
4. <ai> <aii> <aiii> <aiv> <b>
5. < >

Criteria
If 1–4, then criteria met SOCIAL PHO < >

Duration
1. ____________ (years old)
2. < > __________ (years old)
3. < > __________ (months)

*DUR met for SOCIAL PHO < >

Impairment
1. < > home
2. < > school
3. < > peers

SEP ANX	GEN ANX	OCD
1. <a> <b> 2. <a> <b> 3. < > 4. <a> <b> 5. <a> <b> 6. <a> <b> 7. <a> <b> 8. <a> <b>	1. < > ________________ ________________ ________________ ________________ ________________ 2. <a> <b> 3. <a> <b> <c> <d> <e> <f>	A. Compulsions 1. < > ____________ 2. <a> ____________ <b> 3. < > B. Obsessions 1. <a> ____________ <b> ____________ <c> ____________ 2. <a> <b> <c> 3. < > C. Interference 1. <a> <b> <c>
Criteria If ≥3, then criteria met SEP ANX < >	**Criteria** If 1–3, then criteria met GEN ANX < >	**Criteria** If A1, A2, & C, then criteria met Compulsions < > If B1, B2, & C, then criteria met Obsessions < > If Compulsions + and/or Obsessions +, then criteria met OCD < >
Duration 1. __________ (years old) 2. < > ________ (years old) 3. < > ________ (weeks) *DUR met for SEP ANX < >	**Duration** 1. __________ (years old) 2. < > ________ (years old) 3. < > ________ (months) *DUR met for GEN ANX < >	**Duration** 1. __________ (years old) 2. < > ________ (years old) ________ (months) *DUR met for OCD < >
Impairment 1. < > home 2. < > school 3. < > peers	**Impairment** 1. < > home 2. < > school 3. < > peers	**Impairment** 1. < > home 2. < > school 3. < > peers

STRESS (ASD/PTSD)	ANO	BUL
A. Exposure 1. <a> <b> ______________ 2. <a> <b> <c> <d> <e> 3. < > ______________ B. Dissociation 1. <a> <b> <c> <d> 2. < > 3. < > 4. < > 5. < > C. Reexperiencing 1. <a> <b> <c> 2. <a> <b> 3. <a> <b> 4. <a> <b> 5. < > D. Avoidance 1. <a> <b> 2. <a> <b> <c> 3. < > 4. <a> <b> 5. <a> <b> 6. <a> <b> 7. <a> <b> E. Hyperarousal 1. <a> <b> 2. <a> <b> 3. < > 4. < > 5. < >	1. <a> <b> 2. <a> ht: __________ wt: __________ <b> ht: __________ wt: __________ 3. <a> <b> <c> 4. <a> <b> <c> 5. < >	1. < > ______________ ______________ 2. <a> <b> <c> <d> 3. <a> <b> <c> <d> 4. <a> <b>
Criteria If A1 & A2, ≥3 in B, ≥1 in C, ≥3 in D, and ≥2 in E, then criteria met ASD < > If A1 & A2, ≥1 in C, ≥3 in D, and ≥2 in E, then criteria met PTSD < >	**Criteria** If 1–4 (&5 for pubescent girls), then criteria met ANO < >	**Criteria** If 1–4, then criteria met BUL < >
Duration 1. __________ (years old) 2. < > ________ (years old) 3. a. < > ______ (weeks) b. < > c. < > ______ (days) 4. < > ________ (months) *DUR met for ASD < > *DUR met for PTSD < >	**Duration** 1. ________ (years old) 2. < > ______ (years old) 3. < > ______ (months) *DUR met for ANO < >	**Duration** 1. ________ (years old) 2. < > ______ (years old) 3. a. < > _____ (#/week) b. < > _____ (months) *DUR met for BUL < >
Impairment 1. < > home 2. < > school 3. < > peers **Type (PTSD)** Acute < > Regular Onset < > Chronic < > Delayed Onset < >	**Impairment** 1. < > home 2. < > school 3. < > peers	**Impairment** 1. < > home 2. < > school 3. < > peers

DEP/DYS (MDD/DD)

A. Dysphoric Mood
1. <a> <b> <c>
2. <a> <bi> <bii> <biii> <c> <d>

B. Loss of Interest
1. <a> <b>
2. <a> <b> <c>

C. Appetite Changes
1. <a> <b> <c>
2. <a> <b>

D. Sleep Changes

Bedtime: __________

Wakeup: __________

1. <a> <b> <c>
2. <a> <b>

E. Psychomotor Changes
1. <a> <b> <c> <d>
2. <a> <b>

F. Low Energy
1. <a> <b> <c> <d>

G. Guilt
1. <a> <b> <c> <d>
2. <a> <b>

H. Impaired Concentration
1. <a> <b> <c> <d> <e>
2. < >

I. Hopelessness
1. <a> <b> <c>

J. Morbid/Suicidal Thoughts
1. <a> <b>
2. <a> <b> <c> <d> <e>

____

____

____

____

____

DEP/DYS (MDD/DD)

Criteria

If A &/or B & ≥5 of A–H or J,
then criteria met
MDD < >

If A & ≥2 of C, D, F, G, H, or I,
then criteria met
DD < >

Duration
1. ______________ (years old)
2. < > ____________ (years old)
3. MDD < > ________ (weeks)
   DD < > _________ (months)

*DUR met for MDD < >
*DUR met for DD < >

Impairment
1. < > home
2. < > school
3. < > peers

MAN/HYPOMAN

A. Elevated Mood
1. <a> ____________________
   <b> ____________________
   <c> ____________________
2. < > ____________________

B. Other Symptoms
1. <a> ____________________
   <b>
2. <a> <b> <c> ____________
3. <a> <b> <c> <d>
4. <a> <b> <c>
5. < >
6. <a> <b> <c> <d> <e>
7. <a> <b> <c> <d>

C. Interference
1. < >
2. < >

Criteria

If A1(a, b, & c) + ≥3 in B + ≥1 in C
or
A2 + ≥4 in B + ≥1 in C,
then criteria met
MAN < >

If A1(a, b, & c) + ≥3 in B +
none in C
or
A2 + ≥4 in B + none in C,
then criteria met
HYPOMAN < >

Duration
1. ______________ (years old)
2. < > ____________ (years old)
3. MAN < > ________ (weeks)
   HYPO < > _______ (days)

*DUR met for MAN < >
*DUR met for HYPOMAN < >

Impairment
1. < > home
2. < > school
3. < > peers

ENU

1. < >
2. <a> <b>
3. <a> <b>

Criteria

If 1, ≥1 in 2, 3a, and 3b, then criteria met
ENU < >

Duration

1. ____________ (years old)
2. < > _________ (years old)
3. <a> _________ (x/week)
   <b> _________ (months)

*DUR met for ENU < >

Impairment

1. < > home
2. < > school
3. < > peers

Type

Nocturnal	< >
Diurnal	< >
Both	< >

ENC

1. < >
2. < >

Criteria

If both 1 & 2, then criteria met
ENC < >

Duration

1. ____________ (years old)
2. < > _________ (years old)
3. <a> _________ (x/month)
   <b> _________ (months)

*DUR met for ENC < >

Impairment

1. < > home
2. < > school
3. < > peers

SCZ/PSY

A. Psychotic Symptoms
1. <a> <b> <c> <d> <e>
2. <a> <b> <c> <d> <e> <f>
3. < >
4. < >
5. < >

B. Interference
1. < >
2. < >
3. < >

Criteria

If ≥2 in A and ≥1 in B, then criteria met
SCZ < >

If ≥1 in A, then criteria met
PSY < >

Duration

1. ______________ (years old)
2. < > ___________ (years old)
3. < > ___________ (months)

*DUR met for SCZ < >
*DUR met for PSY < >

Impairment

1. < > home
2. < > school
3. < > peers

STRESSORS

A. Child Abuse/Neglect
1. <a> <b> <c>
2. <a> <b> <c> <d>
3. <a> <b> <c> <d>
4. < >
5. < >

Duration

1. ______________________
2. < > ___________________
3. ______________________
4. ______________________
5. < >

B. Other Stressors
1. <a> <b> <c> <d> <e>
2. < >
3. <a> <b>
4. <a> <b> <c>
5. <a> <b>
6. <a> <b>
7. <a> _________________
   <b>
8. <a> <b> <c> <d>
9. < > _________________
   ____
   ____
10. < >
11. < > _________________
   ____
   ____

P-ChIPS Scoring Form
Profile Sheet

Child's Number: ______________________ Date: ______________

Child's Name: ______________________ Time Started: ______________

Date of Birth: ______________ Age: ______________ Time Ended: ______________

Race: ______________ Sex: ______________ Interviewer: ______________

Informant's Name: ______________________

Informant's Relationship (circle one): Mother, Father, Stepmother, Stepfather, Guardian, Other: ______________

	Disorder	Symptoms	Diagnosis	Duration	Clinician's Diagnosis
ADHD	**Attention-Deficit/Hyperactivity Disorder**	<>	<>	<>	**Axis I**
	Type: Inattentive, Hyperactive–Impulsive, Combined				
ODD	**Oppositional Defiant Disorder**	<>	<>	<>	
CD	**Conduct Disorder**	<>	<>	<>	
	Onset: Childhood, Adolescent				
	Severity: Mild, Moderate, Severe				
SUBAB	**Substance Abuse**	<>	<>	<>	
	Substance(s): ______________				
PHO	**Specific Phobia**	<>	<>	<>	**Axis II**
	Type: ______________				
SOCPHO	**Social Phobia**	<>	<>	<>	
SEPANX	**Separation Anxiety Disorder**	<>	<>	<>	**Axis III**
GENANX	**General Anxiety Disorder**	<>	<>	<>	
OCD	**Obsessive-Compulsive Disorder**	<>	<>	<>	
PTSD	**Posttraumatic Stress Disorder**	<>	<>	<>	**Axis IV**
	Type: Acute, Chronic				
	Onset: Regular, Delayed				
ASD	**Acute Stress Disorder**	<>	<>	<>	
ANO	**Anorexia**	<>	<>	<>	**Axis V**
BUL	**Bulimia**	<>	<>	<>	**current:**
DEP	**Major Depressive Disorder**	<>	<>	<>	**past year:**
DYS	**Dysthymic Disorder**	<>	<>	<>	
MAN	**Mania**	<>	<>	<>	
HYPOMAN	**Hypomania**	<>	<>	<>	
ENU	**Enuresis**	<>	<>	<>	
	Type: Nocturnal, Diurnal, Both				
ENC	**Encopresis**	<>	<>	<>	
SCZ	**Schizophrenia**	<>	<>	<>	
PSY	**Psychosis**	<>	<>	<>	

Psychosocial Stressors:

Other Stressors:

Behavioral Observations

Appearance:

Affect:

Effort:

Level of Activity:

Unusual Behaviors:

Presenting Problem

Home

1.

2.

School

1.

2.

3.

4.

5.

Peers/Work

1.

2.

3.

4.

5.

Medication

Type:

Dosage:

Child's Name: ______________________________

Date: ________________

ADHD	ODD	CD
A. Inattention 1. <a> <b> 2. < > 3. <a> <b> 4. <a> <b> <c> 5. < > 6. < > 7. < > 8. <a> <b> 9. <a> <b> B. Hyperactivity–Impulsivity 1. <a> <b> 2. <a> <b> 3. < > 4. <a> <b> 5. < > 6. <a> <b> 7. < > 8. <a> <b> 9. <a> <b> <c>	1. <a> <b> 2. <a> <b> 3. <a> <b> <c> <d> 4. < > 5. <a> <b> 6. < > 7. < > 8. < >	1. < > 2. <a> <b> 3. < > 4. < > 5. < > 6. < > 7. <a> <b> 8. <a> <b> 9. < > 10. <a> <b> 11. < > 12. < > 13. < > 14. < > 15. <a> <b>
Criteria If ≥6 in *A only*, then criteria met Inattentive < > If ≥6 in *B only*, then criteria met Hyperactive–Impulsive < > If ≥6 in A *and* ≥6 in B, then criteria met Combined < >	**Criteria** If ≥4, then criteria met ODD < >	**Criteria** If ≥3, then criteria met CD < >
Duration 1. ____________ (years old) 2. < > _________ (years old) 3. < > __________ (months) * DUR met for ADHD < >	**Duration** 1. ____________ (years old) 2. < > _________ (years old) 3. < > __________ (months) * DUR met for ODD < >	**Duration** 1. ____________ (years old) 2. < > _________ (years old) 3. < > __________ (months) * DUR met for CD < >
Impairment 1. < > home 2. < > school 3. < > peers	**Impairment** 1. < > home 2. < > school 3. < > peers	**Impairment** 1. < > home 2. < > school 3. < > peers **Type** Childhood Onset < > Adolescent Onset < > Mild < > Moderate < > Severe < >

SUB AB

1. < >
   <a>__________
   <b>__________
   <c>__________
   ____
2. < > __________
3. < > __________
4. < > __________

Duration

1. __________ (years old)
2. < > __________ (years old)
   __________ (months)

* DUR met for SUB AB < >

Impairment

1. <a> <b>
2. < >
3. <a> <b>
4. < >

Criteria

If any use (Q1–4) and any impairment (1–4), then criteria met SUB AB < >

Type(s) __________
____
____
____

PHO

1. __________
   ____
   ____
2. <a> <b>
3. <a> <b>
4. <ai> <aii> <aiii> <aiv> <b>
5. <a> <b>

Criteria

If 1–4, then criteria met
PHO < >

Duration

1. __________ (years old)
2. < > __________ (years old)
3. < > __________ (months)

* DUR met for PHO < >

Impairment

1. < > home
2. < > school
3. < > peers

Type(s)

Animal	< >
Natural Environment	< >
Blood–Injection–Injury	< >
Situational	< >
Other __________	< >

SOCIAL PHO

1. <a> <b>
2. < >
3. <a> <b>
4. <ai> <aii> <aiii> <aiv> <b>
5. < >

Criteria

If 1–4, then criteria met
SOCIAL PHO < >

Duration

1. __________ (years old)
2. < > __________ (years old)
3. < > __________ (months)

*DUR met for SOCIAL PHO < >

Impairment

1. < > home
2. < > school
3. < > peers

SEP ANX	GEN ANX	OCD
1. <a> <b> 2. <a> <b> 3. < > 4. <a> <b> 5. <a> <b> 6. <a> <b> 7. <a> <b> 8. <a> <b>	1. < > ____________ ____________ ____________ ____________ ____________ 2. <a> <b> 3. <a> <b> <c> <d> <e> <f>	A. Compulsions 1. < > ____________ 2. <a> ____________ <b> 3. < > B. Obsessions 1. <a> ____________ <b> ____________ <c> ____________ 2. <a> <b> <c> 3. < > C. Interference 1. <a> <b> <c>
Criteria If ≥3, then criteria met SEP ANX < >	**Criteria** If 1–3, then criteria met GEN ANX < >	**Criteria** If A1, A2, & C, then criteria met Compulsions < > If B1, B2, & C, then criteria met Obsessions < > If Compulsions + and/or Obsessions +, then criteria met OCD < >
Duration 1. ____________ (years old) 2. < > __________ (years old) 3. < > __________ (weeks) *DUR met for SEP ANX < >	**Duration** 1. ____________ (years old) 2. < > __________ (years old) 3. < > __________ (months) *DUR met for GEN ANX < >	**Duration** 1. ____________ (years old) 2. < > __________ (years old) __________ (months) *DUR met for OCD < >
Impairment 1. < > home 2. < > school 3. < > peers	**Impairment** 1. < > home 2. < > school 3. < > peers	**Impairment** 1. < > home 2. < > school 3. < > peers

STRESS (ASD/PTSD)	ANO	BUL
A. Exposure 1. <a> <b> ____________ 2. <a> <b> <c> <d> <e> 3. < > ____________ B. Dissociation 1. <a> <b> <c> <d> 2. < > 3. < > 4. < > 5. < > C. Reexperiencing 1. <a> <b> <c> 2. <a> <b> 3. <a> <b> 4. <a> <b> 5. < > D. Avoidance 1. <a> <b> 2. <a> <b> <c> 3. < > 4. <a> <b> 5. <a> <b> 6. <a> <b> 7. <a> <b> E. Hyperarousal 1. <a> <b> 2. <a> <b> 3. < > 4. < > 5. < >	1. <a> <b> 2. <a> ht: ________ wt: ________ <b> ht: ________ wt: ________ 3. <a> <b> <c> 4. <a> <b> <c> 5. < >	1. < > ____________ ____________ 2. <a> <b> <c> <d> 3. <a> <b> <c> <d> 4. <a> <b>
Criteria If A1 & A2, ≥3 in B, ≥1 in C, ≥3 in D, and ≥2 in E, then criteria met ASD < > If A1 & A2, ≥1 in C, ≥3 in D, and ≥2 in E, then criteria met PTSD < >	**Criteria** If 1–4 (&5 for pubescent girls), then criteria met ANO < >	**Criteria** If 1–4, then criteria met BUL < >
Duration 1. ________ (years old) 2. < > ________ (years old) 3. a. < > ______ (weeks) b. < > c. < > ______ (days) 4. < > ________ (months) *DUR met for ASD < > *DUR met for PTSD < >	**Duration** 1. ________ (years old) 2. < > ______ (years old) 3. < > ______ (months) *DUR met for ANO < >	**Duration** 1. ________ (years old) 2. < > ______ (years old) 3. a. < > _____ (#/week) b. < > _____ (months) *DUR met for BUL < >
Impairment 1. < > home 2. < > school 3. < > peers **Type (PTSD)** Acute < > Regular Onset < > Chronic < > Delayed Onset < >	**Impairment** 1. < > home 2. < > school 3. < > peers	**Impairment** 1. < > home 2. < > school 3. < > peers

DEP/DYS (MDD/DD)

A. Dysphoric Mood
1. <a> <b> <c>
2. <a> <bi> <bii> <biii> <c> <d>

B. Loss of Interest
1. <a> <b>
2. <a> <b> <c>

C. Appetite Changes
1. <a> <b> <c>
2. <a> <b>

D. Sleep Changes
Bedtime: ____________
Wakeup: ____________
1. <a> <b> <c>
2. <a> <b>

E. Psychomotor Changes
1. <a> <b> <c> <d>
2. <a> <b>

F. Low Energy
1. <a> <b> <c> <d>

G. Guilt
1. <a> <b> <c> <d>
2. <a> <b>

H. Impaired Concentration
1. <a> <b> <c> <d> <e>
2. < >

I. Hopelessness
1. <a> <b> <c>

J. Morbid/Suicidal Thoughts
1. <a> <b>
2. <a> <b> <c> <d> <e>

____
____
____
____
____

DEP/DYS (MDD/DD)

Criteria

If A &/or B & ≥5 of A–H or J, then criteria met
MDD < >

If A & ≥2 of C, D, F, G, H, or I, then criteria met
DD < >

Duration

1. ______________ (years old)
2. < > ______________ (years old)
3. MDD < > ________ (weeks)
   DD < > ________ (months)

*DUR met for MDD < >
*DUR met for DD < >

Impairment

1. < > home
2. < > school
3. < > peers

MAN/HYPOMAN

A. Elevated Mood
1. <a> ______________________
   <b> ______________________
   <c> ______________________
2. < > ______________________

B. Other Symptoms
1. <a> ______________________
   <b>
2. <a> <b> <c> ____________
3. <a> <b> <c> <d>
4. <a> <b> <c>
5. < >
6. <a> <b> <c> <d> <e>
7. <a> <b> <c> <d>

C. Interference
1. < >
2. < >

Criteria

If A1(a, b, & c) + ≥3 in B + ≥1 in C
or
A2 + ≥4 in B + ≥1 in C, then criteria met
MAN < >

If A1(a, b, & c) + ≥3 in B + none in C
or
A2 + ≥4 in B + none in C, then criteria met
HYPOMAN < >

Duration

1. ______________ (years old)
2. < > ______________ (years old)
3. MAN < > ________ (weeks)
   HYPO < > ________ (days)

*DUR met for MAN < >
*DUR met for HYPOMAN < >

Impairment

1. < > home
2. < > school
3. < > peers

ENU

1. < >
2. <a> <b>
3. <a> <b>

Criteria

If 1, ≥1 in 2, 3a, and 3b, then criteria met
ENU < >

Duration

1. ________ (years old)
2. < > ________ (years old)
3. <a> ________ (x/week)
   <b> ________ (months)

*DUR met for ENU < >

Impairment

1. < > home
2. < > school
3. < > peers

Type

Nocturnal < >
Diurnal < >
Both < >

ENC

1. < >
2. < >

Criteria

If both 1 & 2, then criteria met
ENC < >

Duration

1. ________ (years old)
2. < > ________ (years old)
3. <a> ________ (x/month)
   <b> ________ (months)

*DUR met for ENC < >

Impairment

1. < > home
2. < > school
3. < > peers

SCZ/PSY

A. Psychotic Symptoms
1. <a> <b> <c> <d> <e>
2. <a> <b> <c> <d> <e> <f>
3. < >
4. < >
5. < >

B. Interference
1. < >
2. < >
3. < >

Criteria

If ≥2 in A and ≥1 in B, then criteria met
SCZ < >

If ≥1 in A, then criteria met
PSY < >

Duration

1. ________ (years old)
2. < > ________ (years old)
3. < > ________ (months)

*DUR met for SCZ < >
*DUR met for PSY < >

Impairment

1. < > home
2. < > school
3. < > peers

STRESSORS

A. Child Abuse/Neglect
1. <a> <b> <c>
2. <a> <b> <c> <d>
3. <a> <b> <c> <d>
4. < >
5. < >

Duration

1. ________
2. < > ________
3. ________
4. ________
5. < >

B. Other Stressors
1. <a> <b> <c> <d> <e>
2. < >
3. <a> <b>
4. <a> <b> <c>
5. <a> <b>
6. <a> <b>
7. <a> ________
   <b>
8. <a> <b> <c> <d>
9. < > ________
   ____
   ____
10. < >
11. < > ________
   ____
   ____

P-ChIPS Scoring Form
Profile Sheet

Child's Number: ______________________ Date: ______________

Child's Name: ______________________ Time Started: ______________

Date of Birth: ______________ Age: ______________ Time Ended: ______________

Race: ______________ Sex: ______________ Interviewer: ______________

Informant's Name: ______________________

Informant's Relationship (circle one): Mother, Father, Stepmother, Stepfather, Guardian, Other: ______________

	Disorder	Symptoms	Diagnosis	Duration	Clinician's Diagnosis
ADHD	**Attention-Deficit/Hyperactivity Disorder** *Type:* Inattentive, Hyperactive–Impulsive, Combined	<>	<>	<>	**Axis I**
ODD	**Oppositional Defiant Disorder**	<>	<>	<>	
CD	**Conduct Disorder** *Onset:* Childhood, Adolescent *Severity:* Mild, Moderate, Severe	<>	<>	<>	
SUBAB	**Substance Abuse** *Substance(s):* ____________	<>	<>	<>	
PHO	**Specific Phobia** *Type:* ____________	<>	<>	<>	**Axis II**
SOCPHO	**Social Phobia**	<>	<>	<>	
SEPANX	**Separation Anxiety Disorder**	<>	<>	<>	**Axis III**
GENANX	**General Anxiety Disorder**	<>	<>	<>	
OCD	**Obsessive-Compulsive Disorder**	<>	<>	<>	
PTSD	**Posttraumatic Stress Disorder** *Type:* Acute, Chronic *Onset:* Regular, Delayed	<>	<>	<>	**Axis IV**
ASD	**Acute Stress Disorder**	<>	<>	<>	
ANO	**Anorexia**	<>	<>	<>	**Axis V**
BUL	**Bulimia**	<>	<>	<>	**current:**
DEP	**Major Depressive Disorder**	<>	<>	<>	**past year:**
DYS	**Dysthymic Disorder**	<>	<>	<>	
MAN	**Mania**	<>	<>	<>	
HYPOMAN	**Hypomania**	<>	<>	<>	
ENU	**Enuresis** *Type:* Nocturnal, Diurnal, Both	<>	<>	<>	
ENC	**Encopresis**	<>	<>	<>	
SCZ	**Schizophrenia**	<>	<>	<>	
PSY	**Psychosis**	<>	<>	<>	

Psychosocial Stressors:

Other Stressors:

Behavioral Observations

Appearance:

Affect:

Effort:

Level of Activity:

Unusual Behaviors:

Presenting Problem

Home
1.
2.

School
1.
2.
3.
4.
5.

Peers/Work
1.
2.
3.
4.
5.

Medication
Type:
Dosage:

Child's Name: ______________________

Date: ______________

ADHD	ODD	CD
A. Inattention 1. <a> <b> 2. < > 3. <a> <b> 4. <a> <b> <c> 5. < > 6. < > 7. < > 8. <a> <b> 9. <a> <b> B. Hyperactivity–Impulsivity 1. <a> <b> 2. <a> <b> 3. < > 4. <a> <b> 5. < > 6. <a> <b> 7. < > 8. <a> <b> 9. <a> <b> <c>	1. <a> <b> 2. <a> <b> 3. <a> <b> <c> <d> 4. < > 5. <a> <b> 6. < > 7. < > 8. < >	1. < > 2. <a> <b> 3. < > 4. < > 5. < > 6. < > 7. <a> <b> 8. <a> <b> 9. < > 10. <a> <b> 11. < > 12. < > 13. < > 14. < > 15. <a> <b>
Criteria If ≥6 in *A only*, then criteria met Inattentive < > If ≥6 in *B only*, then criteria met Hyperactive–Impulsive < > If ≥6 in A *and* ≥6 in B, then criteria met Combined < >	**Criteria** If ≥4, then criteria met ODD < >	**Criteria** If ≥3, then criteria met CD < >
Duration 1. __________ (years old) 2. < > ________ (years old) 3. < > _________ (months) * DUR met for ADHD < >	**Duration** 1. __________ (years old) 2. < > ________ (years old) 3. < > _________ (months) * DUR met for ODD < >	**Duration** 1. __________ (years old) 2. < > ________ (years old) 3. < > _________ (months) * DUR met for CD < >
Impairment 1. < > home 2. < > school 3. < > peers	**Impairment** 1. < > home 2. < > school 3. < > peers	**Impairment** 1. < > home 2. < > school 3. < > peers
		Type Childhood Onset < > Adolescent Onset < > Mild < > Moderate < > Severe < >

SUB AB

1. < >
   <a>____________________
   <b>____________________
   <c>____________________
   ____
2. < > ____________________
3. < > ____________________
4. < > ____________________

Duration

1. ____________ (years old)
2. < > __________ (years old)
   __________ (months)

* DUR met for SUB AB < >

Impairment

1. <a> <b>
2. < >
3. <a> <b>
4. < >

Criteria

If any use (Q1–4) and any impairment (1–4), then criteria met SUB AB < >

Type(s) ____________________

____

____

____

PHO

1. ____________________
   ____
   ____
2. <a> <b>
3. <a> <b>
4. <ai> <aii> <aiii> <aiv> <b>
5. <a> <b>

Criteria

If 1–4, then criteria met PHO < >

Duration

1. ____________ (years old)
2. < > __________ (years old)
3. < > __________ (months)

* DUR met for PHO < >

Impairment

1. < > home
2. < > school
3. < > peers

Type(s)

Animal	< >
Natural Environment	< >
Blood–Injection–Injury	< >
Situational	< >
Other ________________	< >

SOCIAL PHO

1. <a> <b>
2. < >
3. <a> <b>
4. <ai> <aii> <aiii> <aiv> <b>
5. < >

Criteria

If 1–4, then criteria met SOCIAL PHO < >

Duration

1. ____________ (years old)
2. < > __________ (years old)
3. < > __________ (months)

*DUR met for SOCIAL PHO < >

Impairment

1. < > home
2. < > school
3. < > peers

SEP ANX	GEN ANX	OCD
1. <a> <b> 2. <a> <b> 3. < > 4. <a> <b> 5. <a> <b> 6. <a> <b> 7. <a> <b> 8. <a> <b>	1. < > ____________ ____________ ____________ ____________ ____________ 2. <a> <b> 3. <a> <b> <c> <d> <e> <f>	A. Compulsions 1. < > ____________ 2. <a> ____________ <b> 3. < > B. Obsessions 1. <a> ____________ <b> ____________ <c> ____________ 2. <a> <b> <c> 3. < > C. Interference 1. <a> <b> <c>
Criteria If ≥3, then criteria met SEP ANX < >	**Criteria** If 1–3, then criteria met GEN ANX < >	**Criteria** If A1, A2, & C, then criteria met Compulsions < > If B1, B2, & C, then criteria met Obsessions < > If Compulsions + and/or Obsessions +, then criteria met OCD < >
Duration 1. ____________ (years old) 2. < > ____________ (years old) 3. < > ____________ (weeks) *DUR met for SEP ANX < >	**Duration** 1. ____________ (years old) 2. < > ____________ (years old) 3. < > ____________ (months) *DUR met for GEN ANX < >	**Duration** 1. ____________ (years old) 2. < > ____________ (years old) ____________ (months) *DUR met for OCD < >
Impairment 1. < > home 2. < > school 3. < > peers	**Impairment** 1. < > home 2. < > school 3. < > peers	**Impairment** 1. < > home 2. < > school 3. < > peers

STRESS (ASD/PTSD)	ANO	BUL
A. Exposure 1. <a> <b> ____________ 2. <a> <b> <c> <d> <e> 3. < > ____________ B. Dissociation 1. <a> <b> <c> <d> 2. < > 3. < > 4. < > 5. < > C. Reexperiencing 1. <a> <b> <c> 2. <a> <b> 3. <a> <b> 4. <a> <b> 5. < > D. Avoidance 1. <a> <b> 2. <a> <b> <c> 3. < > 4. <a> <b> 5. <a> <b> 6. <a> <b> 7. <a> <b> E. Hyperarousal 1. <a> <b> 2. <a> <b> 3. < > 4. < > 5. < >	1. <a> <b> 2. <a> ht: ____________ wt: ____________ <b> ht: ____________ wt: ____________ 3. <a> <b> <c> 4. <a> <b> <c> 5. < >	1. < > ____________ ____________ 2. <a> <b> <c> <d> 3. <a> <b> <c> <d> 4. <a> <b>
Criteria If A1 & A2, ≥3 in B, ≥1 in C, ≥3 in D, and ≥2 in E, then criteria met ASD < > If A1 & A2, ≥1 in C, ≥3 in D, and ≥2 in E, then criteria met PTSD < >	**Criteria** If 1–4 (&5 for pubescent girls), then criteria met ANO < >	**Criteria** If 1–4, then criteria met BUL < >
Duration 1. ____________ (years old) 2. < > ________ (years old) 3. a. < > ______ (weeks) b. < > c. < > ______ (days) 4. < > ________ (months) *DUR met for ASD < > *DUR met for PTSD < >	**Duration** 1. ________ (years old) 2. < > ______ (years old) 3. < > ______ (months) *DUR met for ANO < >	**Duration** 1. ________ (years old) 2. < > ______ (years old) 3. a. < > _____ (#/week) b. < > _____ (months) *DUR met for BUL < >
Impairment 1. < > home 2. < > school 3. < > peers **Type (PTSD)** Acute < > Regular Onset < > Chronic < > Delayed Onset < >	**Impairment** 1. < > home 2. < > school 3. < > peers	**Impairment** 1. < > home 2. < > school 3. < > peers

DEP/DYS (MDD/DD)

A. Dysphoric Mood
1. <a> <b> <c>
2. <a> <bi> <bii> <biii> <c> <d>

B. Loss of Interest
1. <a> <b>
2. <a> <b> <c>

C. Appetite Changes
1. <a> <b> <c>
2. <a> <b>

D. Sleep Changes
Bedtime: __________
Wakeup: __________
1. <a> <b> <c>
2. <a> <b>

E. Psychomotor Changes
1. <a> <b> <c> <d>
2. <a> <b>

F. Low Energy
1. <a> <b> <c> <d>

G. Guilt
1. <a> <b> <c> <d>
2. <a> <b>

H. Impaired Concentration
1. <a> <b> <c> <d> <e>
2. < >

I. Hopelessness
1. <a> <b> <c>

J. Morbid/Suicidal Thoughts
1. <a> <b>
2. <a> <b> <c> <d> <e>

____
____
____
____
____

DEP/DYS (MDD/DD)

Criteria

If A &/or B & ≥5 of A–H or J,
then criteria met
MDD < >

If A & ≥2 of C, D, F, G, H, or I,
then criteria met
DD < >

Duration
1. ______________ (years old)
2. < > ____________ (years old)
3. MDD < > ________ (weeks)
   DD < > ________ (months)

*DUR met for MDD < >
*DUR met for DD < >

Impairment
1. < > home
2. < > school
3. < > peers

MAN/HYPOMAN

A. Elevated Mood
1. <a> ____________________
   <b> ____________________
   <c> ____________________
2. < > ____________________

B. Other Symptoms
1. <a> ____________________
   <b>
2. <a> <b> <c> ____________
3. <a> <b> <c> <d>
4. <a> <b> <c>
5. < >
6. <a> <b> <c> <d> <e>
7. <a> <b> <c> <d>

C. Interference
1. < >
2. < >

Criteria

If A1(a, b, & c) + ≥3 in B + ≥1 in C
or
A2 + ≥4 in B + ≥1 in C,
then criteria met
MAN < >

If A1(a, b, & c) + ≥3 in B +
none in C
or
A2 + ≥4 in B + none in C,
then criteria met
HYPOMAN < >

Duration
1. ______________ (years old)
2. < > ____________ (years old)
3. MAN < > ________ (weeks)
   HYPO < > _______ (days)

*DUR met for MAN < >
*DUR met for HYPOMAN < >

Impairment
1. < > home
2. < > school
3. < > peers

ENU

1. < >
2. <a> <b>
3. <a> <b>

Criteria

If 1, ≥1 in 2, 3a, and 3b,
then criteria met
ENU < >

Duration

1. ____________ (years old)
2. < > __________ (years old)
3. <a> __________ (x/week)
   <b> __________ (months)

*DUR met for ENU < >

Impairment

1. < > home
2. < > school
3. < > peers

Type

Nocturnal	< >
Diurnal	< >
Both	< >

ENC

1. < >
2. < >

Criteria

If both 1 & 2, then criteria met
ENC < >

Duration

1. ____________ (years old)
2. < > __________ (years old)
3. <a> __________ (x/month)
   <b> __________ (months)

*DUR met for ENC < >

Impairment

1. < > home
2. < > school
3. < > peers

SCZ/PSY

A. Psychotic Symptoms

1. <a> <b> <c> <d> <e>
2. <a> <b> <c> <d> <e> <f>
3. < >
4. < >
5. < >

B. Interference

1. < >
2. < >
3. < >

Criteria

If ≥2 in A and ≥1 in B,
then criteria met
SCZ < >

If ≥1 in A, then criteria met
PSY < >

Duration

1. ______________ (years old)
2. < > ____________ (years old)
3. < > ____________ (months)

*DUR met for SCZ < >
*DUR met for PSY < >

Impairment

1. < > home
2. < > school
3. < > peers

STRESSORS

A. Child Abuse/Neglect

1. <a> <b> <c>
2. <a> <b> <c> <d>
3. <a> <b> <c> <d>
4. < >
5. < >

Duration

1. ______________________
2. < > ____________________
3. ______________________
4. ______________________
5. < >

B. Other Stressors

1. <a> <b> <c> <d> <e>
2. < >
3. <a> <b>
4. <a> <b> <c>
5. <a> <b>
6. <a> <b>
7. <a> ________________
   <b>
8. <a> <b> <c> <d>
9. < > ________________
   ____
   ____
10. < >
11. < > ________________
    ____
    ____

P-ChIPS Scoring Form
Profile Sheet

Child's Number: ______________________ Date: ____________

Child's Name: ______________________ Time Started: ____________

Date of Birth: ____________ Age: ____________ Time Ended: ____________

Race: ____________ Sex: ____________ Interviewer: ____________

Informant's Name: ______________________

Informant's Relationship (circle one): Mother, Father, Stepmother, Stepfather, Guardian, Other: ____________

	Disorder	Symptoms	Diagnosis	Duration	Clinician's Diagnosis
ADHD	**Attention-Deficit/Hyperactivity Disorder** *Type:* Inattentive, Hyperactive–Impulsive, Combined	<>	<>	<>	**Axis I**
ODD	**Oppositional Defiant Disorder**	<>	<>	<>	
CD	**Conduct Disorder** *Onset:* Childhood, Adolescent *Severity:* Mild, Moderate, Severe	<>	<>	<>	
SUBAB	**Substance Abuse** *Substance(s):* ____________	<>	<>	<>	
PHO	**Specific Phobia** *Type:* ____________	<>	<>	<>	**Axis II**
SOCPHO	**Social Phobia**	<>	<>	<>	
SEPANX	**Separation Anxiety Disorder**	<>	<>	<>	**Axis III**
GENANX	**General Anxiety Disorder**	<>	<>	<>	
OCD	**Obsessive-Compulsive Disorder**	<>	<>	<>	
PTSD	**Posttraumatic Stress Disorder** *Type:* Acute, Chronic *Onset:* Regular, Delayed	<>	<>	<>	**Axis IV**
ASD	**Acute Stress Disorder**	<>	<>	<>	
ANO	**Anorexia**	<>	<>	<>	**Axis V**
BUL	**Bulimia**	<>	<>	<>	**current:**
DEP	**Major Depressive Disorder**	<>	<>	<>	**past year:**
DYS	**Dysthymic Disorder**	<>	<>	<>	
MAN	**Mania**	<>	<>	<>	
HYPOMAN	**Hypomania**	<>	<>	<>	
ENU	**Enuresis** *Type:* Nocturnal, Diurnal, Both	<>	<>	<>	
ENC	**Encopresis**	<>	<>	<>	
SCZ	**Schizophrenia**	<>	<>	<>	
PSY	**Psychosis**	<>	<>	<>	

Psychosocial Stressors:

Other Stressors:

Behavioral Observations

Appearance:

Affect:

Effort:

Level of Activity:

Unusual Behaviors:

Presenting Problem

Home

1.

2.

School

1.

2.

3.

4.

5.

Peers/Work

1.

2.

3.

4.

5.

Medication

Type:

Dosage:

Child's Name: ____________________

Date: ____________

ADHD	ODD	CD
A. Inattention 1. <a> <b> 2. < > 3. <a> <b> 4. <a> <b> <c> 5. < > 6. < > 7. < > 8. <a> <b> 9. <a> <b> B. Hyperactivity–Impulsivity 1. <a> <b> 2. <a> <b> 3. < > 4. <a> <b> 5. < > 6. <a> <b> 7. < > 8. <a> <b> 9. <a> <b> <c>	1. <a> <b> 2. <a> <b> 3. <a> <b> <c> <d> 4. < > 5. <a> <b> 6. < > 7. < > 8. < >	1. < > 2. <a> <b> 3. < > 4. < > 5. < > 6. < > 7. <a> <b> 8. <a> <b> 9. < > 10. <a> <b> 11. < > 12. < > 13. < > 14. < > 15. <a> <b>
Criteria If ≥6 in *A only*, then criteria met Inattentive < > If ≥6 in *B only*, then criteria met Hyperactive–Impulsive < > If ≥6 in A *and* ≥6 in B, then criteria met Combined < >	**Criteria** If ≥4, then criteria met ODD < >	**Criteria** If ≥3, then criteria met CD < >
Duration 1. __________ (years old) 2. < > ________ (years old) 3. < > ________ (months) * DUR met for ADHD < >	**Duration** 1. __________ (years old) 2. < > ________ (years old) 3. < > ________ (months) * DUR met for ODD < >	**Duration** 1. __________ (years old) 2. < > ________ (years old) 3. < > ________ (months) * DUR met for CD < >
Impairment 1. < > home 2. < > school 3. < > peers	**Impairment** 1. < > home 2. < > school 3. < > peers	**Impairment** 1. < > home 2. < > school 3. < > peers **Type** Childhood Onset < > Adolescent Onset < > Mild < > Moderate < > Severe < >

SUB AB

1. < >
   <a>______________________
   <b>______________________
   <c>______________________
   ____
2. < > ______________________
3. < > ______________________
4. < > ______________________

Duration

1. ______________ (years old)
2. < > __________ (years old)
   __________ (months)

* DUR met for SUB AB < >

Impairment

1. <a> <b>
2. < >
3. <a> <b>
4. < >

Criteria

If any use (Q1–4) and any impairment (1–4), then criteria met SUB AB < >

Type(s) ______________________
____
____
____

PHO

1. ______________________________
   ____
   ____
2. <a> <b>
3. <a> <b>
4. <ai> <aii> <aiii> <aiv> <b>
5. <a> <b>

Criteria

If 1–4, then criteria met PHO < >

Duration

1. ______________ (years old)
2. < > __________ (years old)
3. < > __________ (months)

* DUR met for PHO < >

Impairment

1. < > home
2. < > school
3. < > peers

Type(s)

Animal	< >
Natural Environment	< >
Blood–Injection–Injury	< >
Situational	< >
Other ______________	< >

SOCIAL PHO

1. <a> <b>
2. < >
3. <a> <b>
4. <ai> <aii> <aiii> <aiv> <b>
5. < >

Criteria

If 1–4, then criteria met SOCIAL PHO < >

Duration

1. ______________ (years old)
2. < > __________ (years old)
3. < > __________ (months)

*DUR met for SOCIAL PHO < >

Impairment

1. < > home
2. < > school
3. < > peers

SEP ANX	GEN ANX	OCD
1. <a> <b> 2. <a> <b> 3. < > 4. <a> <b> 5. <a> <b> 6. <a> <b> 7. <a> <b> 8. <a> <b>	1. < > ____________________ ____________________ ____________________ ____________________ ____________________ 2. <a> <b> 3. <a> <b> <c> <d> <e> <f>	A. Compulsions 1. < > ______________ 2. <a> ______________ <b> 3. < > B. Obsessions 1. <a> ______________ <b> ______________ <c> ______________ 2. <a> <b> <c> 3. < > C. Interference 1. <a> <b> <c>
Criteria If ≥3, then criteria met SEP ANX < >	**Criteria** If 1–3, then criteria met GEN ANX < >	**Criteria** If A1, A2, & C, then criteria met Compulsions < > If B1, B2, & C, then criteria met Obsessions < > If Compulsions + and/or Obsessions +, then criteria met OCD < >
Duration 1. ____________ (years old) 2. < > __________ (years old) 3. < > __________ (weeks) *DUR met for SEP ANX < >	**Duration** 1. ____________ (years old) 2. < > __________ (years old) 3. < > __________ (months) *DUR met for GEN ANX < >	**Duration** 1. ____________ (years old) 2. < > __________ (years old) __________ (months) *DUR met for OCD < >
Impairment 1. < > home 2. < > school 3. < > peers	**Impairment** 1. < > home 2. < > school 3. < > peers	**Impairment** 1. < > home 2. < > school 3. < > peers

STRESS (ASD/PTSD)

A. Exposure
1. <a> <b> ________________
2. <a> <b> <c> <d> <e>
3. < > ________________

B. Dissociation
1. <a> <b> <c> <d>
2. < >
3. < >
4. < >
5. < >

C. Reexperiencing
1. <a> <b> <c>
2. <a> <b>
3. <a> <b>
4. <a> <b>
5. < >

D. Avoidance
1. <a> <b>
2. <a> <b> <c>
3. < >
4. <a> <b>
5. <a> <b>
6. <a> <b>
7. <a> <b>

E. Hyperarousal
1. <a> <b>
2. <a> <b>
3. < >
4. < >
5. < >

Criteria

If A1 & A2, ≥3 in B, ≥1 in C, ≥3 in D, and ≥2 in E, then criteria met ASD < >

If A1 & A2, ≥1 in C, ≥3 in D, and ≥2 in E, then criteria met PTSD < >

Duration
1. ____________ (years old)
2. < > ____________ (years old)
3. a. < > ________ (weeks)
   b. < >
   c. < > ________ (days)
4. < > ____________ (months)

*DUR met for ASD < >
*DUR met for PTSD < >

Impairment
1. < > home
2. < > school
3. < > peers

Type (PTSD)

Acute < > Regular Onset < >
Chronic < > Delayed Onset < >

ANO

1. <a> <b>
2. <a>
   ht: ____________
   wt: ____________
   <b>
   ht: ____________
   wt: ____________
3. <a> <b> <c>
4. <a> <b> <c>
5. < >

Criteria

If 1–4 (&5 for pubescent girls), then criteria met ANO < >

Duration
1. ____________ (years old)
2. < > ________ (years old)
3. < > ________ (months)

*DUR met for ANO < >

Impairment
1. < > home
2. < > school
3. < > peers

BUL

1. < > ________________
____
2. <a> <b> <c> <d>
3. <a> <b> <c> <d>
4. <a> <b>

Criteria

If 1–4, then criteria met BUL < >

Duration
1. ____________ (years old)
2. < > ________ (years old)
3. a. < > ______ (#/week)
   b. < > ______ (months)

*DUR met for BUL < >

Impairment
1. < > home
2. < > school
3. < > peers

DEP/DYS (MDD/DD)

A. Dysphoric Mood
- 1. <a> <b> <c>
- 2. <a> <bi> <bii> <biii> <c> <d>

B. Loss of Interest
- 1. <a> <b>
- 2. <a> <b> <c>

C. Appetite Changes
- 1. <a> <b> <c>
- 2. <a> <b>

D. Sleep Changes
- Bedtime: ______
- Wakeup: ______
- 1. <a> <b> <c>
- 2. <a> <b>

E. Psychomotor Changes
- 1. <a> <b> <c> <d>
- 2. <a> <b>

F. Low Energy
- 1. <a> <b> <c> <d>

G. Guilt
- 1. <a> <b> <c> <d>
- 2. <a> <b>

H. Impaired Concentration
- 1. <a> <b> <c> <d> <e>
- 2. < >

I. Hopelessness
- 1. <a> <b> <c>

J. Morbid/Suicidal Thoughts
- 1. <a> <b>
- 2. <a> <b> <c> <d> <e>

______
______
______
______
______

DEP/DYS (MDD/DD)

Criteria

If A &/or B & ≥5 of A–H or J, then criteria met MDD < >

If A & ≥2 of C, D, F, G, H, or I, then criteria met DD < >

Duration
1. ______ (years old)
2. < > ______ (years old)
3. MDD < > ______ (weeks)
   DD < > ______ (months)

*DUR met for MDD < >
*DUR met for DD < >

Impairment
1. < > home
2. < > school
3. < > peers

MAN/HYPOMAN

A. Elevated Mood
- 1. <a> ______
  <b> ______
  <c> ______
- 2. < > ______

B. Other Symptoms
- 1. <a> ______
  <b>
- 2. <a> <b> <c> ______
- 3. <a> <b> <c> <d>
- 4. <a> <b> <c>
- 5. < >
- 6. <a> <b> <c> <d> <e>
- 7. <a> <b> <c> <d>

C. Interference
- 1. < >
- 2. < >

Criteria

If A1(a, b, & c) + ≥3 in B + ≥1 in C *or* A2 + ≥4 in B + ≥1 in C, then criteria met MAN < >

If A1(a, b, & c) + ≥3 in B + none in C *or* A2 + ≥4 in B + none in C, then criteria met HYPOMAN < >

Duration
1. ______ (years old)
2. < > ______ (years old)
3. MAN < > ______ (weeks)
   HYPO < > ______ (days)

*DUR met for MAN < >
*DUR met for HYPOMAN < >

Impairment
1. < > home
2. < > school
3. < > peers

ENU

1. < >
2. <a> <b>
3. <a> <b>

Criteria

If 1, ≥1 in 2, 3a, and 3b, then criteria met

ENU < >

Duration

1. ______ (years old)
2. < > ______ (years old)
3. <a> ______ (x/week)
   <b> ______ (months)

*DUR met for ENU < >

Impairment

1. < > home
2. < > school
3. < > peers

Type

Nocturnal < >
Diurnal < >
Both < >

ENC

1. < >
2. < >

Criteria

If both 1 & 2, then criteria met

ENC < >

Duration

1. ______ (years old)
2. < > ______ (years old)
3. <a> ______ (x/month)
   <b> ______ (months)

*DUR met for ENC < >

Impairment

1. < > home
2. < > school
3. < > peers

SCZ/PSY

A. Psychotic Symptoms
1. <a> <b> <c> <d> <e>
2. <a> <b> <c> <d> <e> <f>
3. < >
4. < >
5. < >

B. Interference
1. < >
2. < >
3. < >

Criteria

If ≥2 in A and ≥1 in B, then criteria met

SCZ < >

If ≥1 in A, then criteria met

PSY < >

Duration

1. ______ (years old)
2. < > ______ (years old)
3. < > ______ (months)

*DUR met for SCZ < >

*DUR met for PSY < >

Impairment

1. < > home
2. < > school
3. < > peers

STRESSORS

A. Child Abuse/Neglect
1. <a> <b> <c>
2. <a> <b> <c> <d>
3. <a> <b> <c> <d>
4. < >
5. < >

Duration

1. ______
2. < > ______
3. ______
4. ______
5. < >

B. Other Stressors
1. <a> <b> <c> <d> <e>
2. < >
3. <a> <b>
4. <a> <b> <c>
5. <a> <b>
6. <a> <b>
7. <a> ______
   <b>
8. <a> <b> <c> <d>
9. < > ______
   ______
   ______
10. < >
11. < > ______
    ______
    ______

P-ChIPS Scoring Form
Profile Sheet

Child's Number: ______________________ Date: ______________

Child's Name: ______________________ Time Started: ______________

Date of Birth: ______________ Age: ______________ Time Ended: ______________

Race: ______________ Sex: ______________ Interviewer: ______________

Informant's Name: ______________________

Informant's Relationship (circle one): Mother, Father, Stepmother, Stepfather, Guardian, Other: ______________

	Disorder	Symptoms	Diagnosis	Duration	Clinician's Diagnosis
ADHD	**Attention-Deficit/Hyperactivity Disorder**	<>	<>	<>	**Axis I**
	Type: Inattentive, Hyperactive–Impulsive, Combined				
ODD	**Oppositional Defiant Disorder**	<>	<>	<>	
CD	**Conduct Disorder**	<>	<>	<>	
	Onset: Childhood, Adolescent				
	Severity: Mild, Moderate, Severe				
SUBAB	**Substance Abuse**	<>	<>	<>	
	Substance(s): ______________				
PHO	**Specific Phobia**	<>	<>	<>	**Axis II**
	Type: ______________				
SOCPHO	**Social Phobia**	<>	<>	<>	
SEPANX	**Separation Anxiety Disorder**	<>	<>	<>	**Axis III**
GENANX	**General Anxiety Disorder**	<>	<>	<>	
OCD	**Obsessive-Compulsive Disorder**	<>	<>	<>	
PTSD	**Posttraumatic Stress Disorder**	<>	<>	<>	**Axis IV**
	Type: Acute, Chronic				
	Onset: Regular, Delayed				
ASD	**Acute Stress Disorder**	<>	<>	<>	
ANO	**Anorexia**	<>	<>	<>	**Axis V**
BUL	**Bulimia**	<>	<>	<>	**current:**
DEP	**Major Depressive Disorder**	<>	<>	<>	**past year:**
DYS	**Dysthymic Disorder**	<>	<>	<>	
MAN	**Mania**	<>	<>	<>	
HYPOMAN	**Hypomania**	<>	<>	<>	
ENU	**Enuresis**	<>	<>	<>	
	Type: Nocturnal, Diurnal, Both				
ENC	**Encopresis**	<>	<>	<>	
SCZ	**Schizophrenia**	<>	<>	<>	
PSY	**Psychosis**	<>	<>	<>	

Psychosocial Stressors:

Other Stressors:

Behavioral Observations

Appearance:

Affect:

Effort:

Level of Activity:

Unusual Behaviors:

Presenting Problem

Home

1.

2.

School

1.

2.

3.

4.

5.

Peers/Work

1.

2.

3.

4.

5.

Medication

Type:

Dosage:

Child's Name: ____________________

Date: ____________

ADHD	ODD	CD
A. Inattention 1. <a> <b> 2. < > 3. <a> <b> 4. <a> <b> <c> 5. < > 6. < > 7. < > 8. <a> <b> 9. <a> <b> B. Hyperactivity–Impulsivity 1. <a> <b> 2. <a> <b> 3. < > 4. <a> <b> 5. < > 6. <a> <b> 7. < > 8. <a> <b> 9. <a> <b> <c>	1. <a> <b> 2. <a> <b> 3. <a> <b> <c> <d> 4. < > 5. <a> <b> 6. < > 7. < > 8. < >	1. < > 2. <a> <b> 3. < > 4. < > 5. < > 6. < > 7. <a> <b> 8. <a> <b> 9. < > 10. <a> <b> 11. < > 12. < > 13. < > 14. < > 15. <a> <b>
Criteria If $\geq$6 in *A only*, then criteria met Inattentive < > If $\geq$6 in *B only*, then criteria met Hyperactive–Impulsive < > If $\geq$6 in A *and* $\geq$6 in B, then criteria met Combined < >	**Criteria** If $\geq$4, then criteria met ODD < >	**Criteria** If $\geq$3, then criteria met CD < >
Duration 1. ________ (years old) 2. < > ______ (years old) 3. < > ______ (months) * DUR met for ADHD < >	**Duration** 1. ________ (years old) 2. < > ______ (years old) 3. < > ______ (months) * DUR met for ODD < >	**Duration** 1. ________ (years old) 2. < > ______ (years old) 3. < > ______ (months) * DUR met for CD < >
Impairment 1. < > home 2. < > school 3. < > peers	**Impairment** 1. < > home 2. < > school 3. < > peers	**Impairment** 1. < > home 2. < > school 3. < > peers **Type** Childhood Onset < > Adolescent Onset < > Mild < > Moderate < > Severe < >

SUB AB

1. < >
   <a>____________________
   <b>____________________
   <c>____________________
   ____
2. < > ____________________
3. < > ____________________
4. < > ____________________

Duration

1. ____________ (years old)
2. < > __________ (years old)
   __________ (months)

* DUR met for SUB AB < >

Impairment

1. <a> <b>
2. < >
3. <a> <b>
4. < >

Criteria

If any use (Q1–4) and any impairment (1–4), then criteria met SUB AB < >

Type(s) ____________________

____

____

____

PHO

1. ____________________
   ____
   ____
2. <a> <b>
3. <a> <b>
4. <ai> <aii> <aiii> <aiv> <b>
5. <a> <b>

Criteria

If 1–4, then criteria met PHO < >

Duration

1. ____________ (years old)
2. < > __________ (years old)
3. < > __________ (months)

* DUR met for PHO < >

Impairment

1. < > home
2. < > school
3. < > peers

Type(s)

Animal	< >
Natural Environment	< >
Blood–Injection–Injury	< >
Situational	< >
Other ________________	< >

SOCIAL PHO

1. <a> <b>
2. < >
3. <a> <b>
4. <ai> <aii> <aiii> <aiv> <b>
5. < >

Criteria

If 1–4, then criteria met SOCIAL PHO < >

Duration

1. ____________ (years old)
2. < > __________ (years old)
3. < > __________ (months)

*DUR met for SOCIAL PHO < >

Impairment

1. < > home
2. < > school
3. < > peers

SEP ANX	GEN ANX	OCD
1. <a> <b> 2. <a> <b> 3. < > 4. <a> <b> 5. <a> <b> 6. <a> <b> 7. <a> <b> 8. <a> <b>	1. < > ____________ ____________ ____________ ____________ ____________ 2. <a> <b> 3. <a> <b> <c> <d> <e> <f>	A. Compulsions 1. < > ____________ 2. <a> ____________ <b> 3. < > B. Obsessions 1. <a> ____________ <b> ____________ <c> ____________ 2. <a> <b> <c> 3. < > C. Interference 1. <a> <b> <c>
Criteria If ≥3, then criteria met SEP ANX < >	**Criteria** If 1–3, then criteria met GEN ANX < >	**Criteria** If A1, A2, & C, then criteria met Compulsions < > If B1, B2, & C, then criteria met Obsessions < > If Compulsions + and/or Obsessions +, then criteria met OCD < >
Duration 1. ____________ (years old) 2. < > ____________ (years old) 3. < > ____________ (weeks) *DUR met for SEP ANX < >	**Duration** 1. ____________ (years old) 2. < > ____________ (years old) 3. < > ____________ (months) *DUR met for GEN ANX < >	**Duration** 1. ____________ (years old) 2. < > ____________ (years old) ____________ (months) *DUR met for OCD < >
Impairment 1. < > home 2. < > school 3. < > peers	**Impairment** 1. < > home 2. < > school 3. < > peers	**Impairment** 1. < > home 2. < > school 3. < > peers

STRESS (ASD/PTSD)	ANO	BUL
A. Exposure 1. <a> <b> ____________ 2. <a> <b> <c> <d> <e> 3. < > ____________ B. Dissociation 1. <a> <b> <c> <d> 2. < > 3. < > 4. < > 5. < > C. Reexperiencing 1. <a> <b> <c> 2. <a> <b> 3. <a> <b> 4. <a> <b> 5. < > D. Avoidance 1. <a> <b> 2. <a> <b> <c> 3. < > 4. <a> <b> 5. <a> <b> 6. <a> <b> 7. <a> <b> E. Hyperarousal 1. <a> <b> 2. <a> <b> 3. < > 4. < > 5. < >	1. <a> <b> 2. <a> ht: ____________ wt: ____________ <b> ht: ____________ wt: ____________ 3. <a> <b> <c> 4. <a> <b> <c> 5. < >	1. < > ____________ ____________ 2. <a> <b> <c> <d> 3. <a> <b> <c> <d> 4. <a> <b>
Criteria If A1 & A2, ≥3 in B, ≥1 in C, ≥3 in D, and ≥2 in E, then criteria met ASD < > If A1 & A2, ≥1 in C, ≥3 in D, and ≥2 in E, then criteria met PTSD < >	**Criteria** If 1–4 (&5 for pubescent girls), then criteria met ANO < >	**Criteria** If 1–4, then criteria met BUL < >
Duration 1. ____________ (years old) 2. < > ____________ (years old) 3. a. < > ________ (weeks) b. < > c. < > ________ (days) 4. < > ____________ (months) *DUR met for ASD < > *DUR met for PTSD < >	**Duration** 1. ____________ (years old) 2. < > ________ (years old) 3. < > ________ (months) *DUR met for ANO < >	**Duration** 1. ____________ (years old) 2. < > ________ (years old) 3. a. < > ______ (#/week) b. < > ______ (months) *DUR met for BUL < >
Impairment 1. < > home 2. < > school 3. < > peers **Type (PTSD)** Acute < > Regular Onset < > Chronic < > Delayed Onset < >	**Impairment** 1. < > home 2. < > school 3. < > peers	**Impairment** 1. < > home 2. < > school 3. < > peers

DEP/DYS (MDD/DD)

A. Dysphoric Mood
1. <a> <b> <c>
2. <a> <bi> <bii> <biii> <c> <d>

B. Loss of Interest
1. <a> <b>
2. <a> <b> <c>

C. Appetite Changes
1. <a> <b> <c>
2. <a> <b>

D. Sleep Changes
Bedtime: ____________
Wakeup: ____________
1. <a> <b> <c>
2. <a> <b>

E. Psychomotor Changes
1. <a> <b> <c> <d>
2. <a> <b>

F. Low Energy
1. <a> <b> <c> <d>

G. Guilt
1. <a> <b> <c> <d>
2. <a> <b>

H. Impaired Concentration
1. <a> <b> <c> <d> <e>
2. < >

I. Hopelessness
1. <a> <b> <c>

J. Morbid/Suicidal Thoughts
1. <a> <b>
2. <a> <b> <c> <d> <e>

____
____
____
____
____

DEP/DYS (MDD/DD)

Criteria

If A &/or B & ≥5 of A–H or J, then criteria met
MDD < >

If A & ≥2 of C, D, F, G, H, or I, then criteria met
DD < >

Duration
1. ____________ (years old)
2. < > ____________ (years old)
3. MDD < > ________ (weeks)
DD < > ________ (months)

*DUR met for MDD < >
*DUR met for DD < >

Impairment
1. < > home
2. < > school
3. < > peers

MAN/HYPOMAN

A. Elevated Mood
1. <a> ____________________
<b> ____________________
<c> ____________________
2. < > ____________________

B. Other Symptoms
1. <a> ____________________
<b>
2. <a> <b> <c> ____________
3. <a> <b> <c> <d>
4. <a> <b> <c>
5. < >
6. <a> <b> <c> <d> <e>
7. <a> <b> <c> <d>

C. Interference
1. < >
2. < >

Criteria

If A1(a, b, & c) + ≥3 in B + ≥1 in C
or
A2 + ≥4 in B + ≥1 in C, then criteria met
MAN < >

If A1(a, b, & c) + ≥3 in B + none in C
or
A2 + ≥4 in B + none in C, then criteria met
HYPOMAN < >

Duration
1. ____________ (years old)
2. < > ____________ (years old)
3. MAN < > ________ (weeks)
HYPO < > ________ (days)

*DUR met for MAN < >
*DUR met for HYPOMAN < >

Impairment
1. < > home
2. < > school
3. < > peers

ENU

1. < >
2. <a> <b>
3. <a> <b>

Criteria

If 1, ≥1 in 2, 3a, and 3b, then criteria met

ENU < >

Duration

1. ____________ (years old)
2. < > __________ (years old)
3. <a> __________ (x/week)
   <b> __________ (months)

*DUR met for ENU < >

Impairment

1. < > home
2. < > school
3. < > peers

Type

Nocturnal	< >
Diurnal	< >
Both	< >

ENC

1. < >
2. < >

Criteria

If both 1 & 2, then criteria met

ENC < >

Duration

1. ____________ (years old)
2. < > __________ (years old)
3. <a> __________ (x/month)
   <b> __________ (months)

*DUR met for ENC < >

Impairment

1. < > home
2. < > school
3. < > peers

SCZ/PSY

A. Psychotic Symptoms

1. <a> <b> <c> <d> <e>
2. <a> <b> <c> <d> <e> <f>
3. < >
4. < >
5. < >

B. Interference

1. < >
2. < >
3. < >

Criteria

If ≥2 in A and ≥1 in B, then criteria met

SCZ < >

If ≥1 in A, then criteria met

PSY < >

Duration

1. ______________ (years old)
2. < > ___________ (years old)
3. < > ___________ (months)

*DUR met for SCZ < >

*DUR met for PSY < >

Impairment

1. < > home
2. < > school
3. < > peers

STRESSORS

A. Child Abuse/Neglect

1. <a> <b> <c>
2. <a> <b> <c> <d>
3. <a> <b> <c> <d>
4. < >
5. < >

Duration

1. ______________________
2. < > ___________________
3. ______________________
4. ______________________
5. < >

B. Other Stressors

1. <a> <b> <c> <d> <e>
2. < >
3. <a> <b>
4. <a> <b> <c>
5. <a> <b>
6. <a> <b>
7. <a> ________________
   <b>
8. <a> <b> <c> <d>
9. < > ________________
   ____
   ____
10. < >
11. < > ________________
    ____
    ____

P-ChIPS Scoring Form
Profile Sheet

Child's Number: ______________________ Date: ______________

Child's Name: ______________________ Time Started: ______________

Date of Birth: ______________ Age: ______________ Time Ended: ______________

Race: ______________ Sex: ______________ Interviewer: ______________

Informant's Name: ______________________

Informant's Relationship (circle one): Mother, Father, Stepmother, Stepfather, Guardian, Other: ______________

	Disorder	Symptoms	Diagnosis	Duration	Clinician's Diagnosis
ADHD	**Attention-Deficit/Hyperactivity Disorder** *Type:* Inattentive, Hyperactive–Impulsive, Combined	<>	<>	<>	**Axis I**
ODD	**Oppositional Defiant Disorder**	<>	<>	<>	
CD	**Conduct Disorder** *Onset:* Childhood, Adolescent *Severity:* Mild, Moderate, Severe	<>	<>	<>	
SUBAB	**Substance Abuse** *Substance(s):* ______________	<>	<>	<>	
PHO	**Specific Phobia** *Type:* ______________	<>	<>	<>	**Axis II**
SOCPHO	**Social Phobia**	<>	<>	<>	
SEPANX	**Separation Anxiety Disorder**	<>	<>	<>	**Axis III**
GENANX	**General Anxiety Disorder**	<>	<>	<>	
OCD	**Obsessive-Compulsive Disorder**	<>	<>	<>	
PTSD	**Posttraumatic Stress Disorder** *Type:* Acute, Chronic *Onset:* Regular, Delayed	<>	<>	<>	**Axis IV**
ASD	**Acute Stress Disorder**	<>	<>	<>	
ANO	**Anorexia**	<>	<>	<>	**Axis V**
BUL	**Bulimia**	<>	<>	<>	**current:**
DEP	**Major Depressive Disorder**	<>	<>	<>	**past year:**
DYS	**Dysthymic Disorder**	<>	<>	<>	
MAN	**Mania**	<>	<>	<>	
HYPOMAN	**Hypomania**	<>	<>	<>	
ENU	**Enuresis** *Type:* Nocturnal, Diurnal, Both	<>	<>	<>	
ENC	**Encopresis**	<>	<>	<>	
SCZ	**Schizophrenia**	<>	<>	<>	
PSY	**Psychosis**	<>	<>	<>	

Psychosocial Stressors:

Other Stressors:

Behavioral Observations

Appearance:

Affect:

Effort:

Level of Activity:

Unusual Behaviors:

Presenting Problem

Home

1.

2.

School

1.

2.

3.

4.

5.

Peers/Work

1.

2.

3.

4.

5.

Medication

Type:

Dosage:

Child's Name: ____________________

Date: ____________

ADHD	ODD	CD
A. Inattention 1. <a> <b> 2. < > 3. <a> <b> 4. <a> <b> <c> 5. < > 6. < > 7. < > 8. <a> <b> 9. <a> <b> B. Hyperactivity–Impulsivity 1. <a> <b> 2. <a> <b> 3. < > 4. <a> <b> 5. < > 6. <a> <b> 7. < > 8. <a> <b> 9. <a> <b> <c>	1. <a> <b> 2. <a> <b> 3. <a> <b> <c> <d> 4. < > 5. <a> <b> 6. < > 7. < > 8. < >	1. < > 2. <a> <b> 3. < > 4. < > 5. < > 6. < > 7. <a> <b> 8. <a> <b> 9. < > 10. <a> <b> 11. < > 12. < > 13. < > 14. < > 15. <a> <b>
Criteria If ≥6 in *A only*, then criteria met Inattentive < > If ≥6 in *B only*, then criteria met Hyperactive–Impulsive < > If ≥6 in A *and* ≥6 in B, then criteria met Combined < >	**Criteria** If ≥4, then criteria met ODD < >	**Criteria** If ≥3, then criteria met CD < >
Duration 1. ________ (years old) 2. < > ________ (years old) 3. < > ________ (months) * DUR met for ADHD < >	**Duration** 1. ________ (years old) 2. < > ________ (years old) 3. < > ________ (months) * DUR met for ODD < >	**Duration** 1. ________ (years old) 2. < > ________ (years old) 3. < > ________ (months) * DUR met for CD < >
Impairment 1. < > home 2. < > school 3. < > peers	**Impairment** 1. < > home 2. < > school 3. < > peers	**Impairment** 1. < > home 2. < > school 3. < > peers **Type** Childhood Onset < > Adolescent Onset < > Mild < > Moderate < > Severe < >

SUB AB

1. < >
   <a>____________________
   <b>____________________
   <c>____________________
   ____
2. < > ____________________
3. < > ____________________
4. < > ____________________

Duration

1. ____________ (years old)
2. < > __________ (years old)
   __________ (months)

* DUR met for SUB AB < >

Impairment

1. <a> <b>
2. < >
3. <a> <b>
4. < >

Criteria

If any use (Q1–4) and any impairment (1–4), then criteria met SUB AB < >

Type(s) ____________________

____

____

____

PHO

1. ____________________
   ____
   ____
2. <a> <b>
3. <a> <b>
4. <ai> <aii> <aiii> <aiv> <b>
5. <a> <b>

Criteria

If 1–4, then criteria met PHO < >

Duration

1. ____________ (years old)
2. < > __________ (years old)
3. < > __________ (months)

* DUR met for PHO < >

Impairment

1. < > home
2. < > school
3. < > peers

Type(s)

Animal	< >
Natural Environment	< >
Blood–Injection–Injury	< >
Situational	< >
Other ____________________	< >

SOCIAL PHO

1. <a> <b>
2. < >
3. <a> <b>
4. <ai> <aii> <aiii> <aiv> <b>
5. < >

Criteria

If 1–4, then criteria met SOCIAL PHO < >

Duration

1. ____________ (years old)
2. < > __________ (years old)
3. < > __________ (months)

*DUR met for SOCIAL PHO < >

Impairment

1. < > home
2. < > school
3. < > peers

SEP ANX	GEN ANX	OCD
1. <a> <b> 2. <a> <b> 3. < > 4. <a> <b> 5. <a> <b> 6. <a> <b> 7. <a> <b> 8. <a> <b>	1. < > ______________ ______________ ______________ ______________ ______________ 2. <a> <b> 3. <a> <b> <c> <d> <e> <f>	A. Compulsions 1. < > ______________ 2. <a> ______________ <b> 3. < > B. Obsessions 1. <a> ______________ <b> ______________ <c> ______________ 2. <a> <b> <c> 3. < > C. Interference 1. <a> <b> <c>
Criteria If ≥3, then criteria met SEP ANX < >	**Criteria** If 1–3, then criteria met GEN ANX < >	**Criteria** If A1, A2, & C, then criteria met Compulsions < > If B1, B2, & C, then criteria met Obsessions < > If Compulsions + and/or Obsessions +, then criteria met OCD < >
Duration 1. ______________ (years old) 2. < > ___________ (years old) 3. < > ___________ (weeks) *DUR met for SEP ANX < >	**Duration** 1. ______________ (years old) 2. < > ___________ (years old) 3. < > ___________ (months) *DUR met for GEN ANX < >	**Duration** 1. ______________ (years old) 2. < > ___________ (years old) ___________ (months) *DUR met for OCD < >
Impairment 1. < > home 2. < > school 3. < > peers	**Impairment** 1. < > home 2. < > school 3. < > peers	**Impairment** 1. < > home 2. < > school 3. < > peers

STRESS (ASD/PTSD)

A. Exposure
1. <a> <b> ____________________
2. <a> <b> <c> <d> <e>
3. < > ____________________

B. Dissociation
1. <a> <b> <c> <d>
2. < >
3. < >
4. < >
5. < >

C. Reexperiencing
1. <a> <b> <c>
2. <a> <b>
3. <a> <b>
4. <a> <b>
5. < >

D. Avoidance
1. <a> <b>
2. <a> <b> <c>
3. < >
4. <a> <b>
5. <a> <b>
6. <a> <b>
7. <a> <b>

E. Hyperarousal
1. <a> <b>
2. <a> <b>
3. < >
4. < >
5. < >

Criteria

If A1 & A2, ≥3 in B, ≥1 in C, ≥3 in D, and ≥2 in E, then criteria met ASD < >

If A1 & A2, ≥1 in C, ≥3 in D, and ≥2 in E, then criteria met PTSD < >

Duration
1. ____________ (years old)
2. < > ____________ (years old)
3. a. < > ________ (weeks)
   b. < >
   c. < > ________ (days)
4. < > ____________ (months)

*DUR met for ASD < >
*DUR met for PTSD < >

Impairment
1. < > home
2. < > school
3. < > peers

Type (PTSD)

Acute < > Regular Onset < >
Chronic < > Delayed Onset < >

ANO

1. <a> <b>
2. <a>
   ht: ______________
   wt: ______________
   <b>
   ht: ______________
   wt: ______________
3. <a> <b> <c>
4. <a> <b> <c>
5. < >

Criteria

If 1–4 (&5 for pubescent girls), then criteria met ANO < >

Duration
1. ___________ (years old)
2. < > ________ (years old)
3. < > ________ (months)

*DUR met for ANO < >

Impairment
1. < > home
2. < > school
3. < > peers

BUL

1. < > ____________________
____
2. <a> <b> <c> <d>
3. <a> <b> <c> <d>
4. <a> <b>

Criteria

If 1–4, then criteria met BUL < >

Duration
1. ___________ (years old)
2. < > ________ (years old)
3. a. < > ______ (#/week)
   b. < > ______ (months)

*DUR met for BUL < >

Impairment
1. < > home
2. < > school
3. < > peers

DEP/DYS (MDD/DD)

A. Dysphoric Mood
   1. <a> <b> <c>
   2. <a> <bi> <bii> <biii> <c> <d>

B. Loss of Interest
   1. <a> <b>
   2. <a> <b> <c>

C. Appetite Changes
   1. <a> <b> <c>
   2. <a> <b>

D. Sleep Changes
   Bedtime: __________
   Wakeup: __________
   1. <a> <b> <c>
   2. <a> <b>

E. Psychomotor Changes
   1. <a> <b> <c> <d>
   2. <a> <b>

F. Low Energy
   1. <a> <b> <c> <d>

G. Guilt
   1. <a> <b> <c> <d>
   2. <a> <b>

H. Impaired Concentration
   1. <a> <b> <c> <d> <e>
   2. < >

I. Hopelessness
   1. <a> <b> <c>

J. Morbid/Suicidal Thoughts
   1. <a> <b>
   2. <a> <b> <c> <d> <e>

____
____
____
____
____

DEP/DYS (MDD/DD)

Criteria

If A &/or B & ≥5 of A–H or J,
then criteria met
MDD < >

If A & ≥2 of C, D, F, G, H, or I,
then criteria met
DD < >

Duration

1. ______________ (years old)
2. < > ____________ (years old)
3. MDD < > ________ (weeks)
   DD < > _________ (months)

*DUR met for MDD < >
*DUR met for DD < >

Impairment

1. < > home
2. < > school
3. < > peers

MAN/HYPOMAN

A. Elevated Mood
   1. <a> ______________________
      <b> ______________________
      <c> ______________________
   2. < > ______________________

B. Other Symptoms
   1. <a> ______________________
      <b>
   2. <a> <b> <c> ____________
   3. <a> <b> <c> <d>
   4. <a> <b> <c>
   5. < >
   6. <a> <b> <c> <d> <e>
   7. <a> <b> <c> <d>

C. Interference
   1. < >
   2. < >

Criteria

If A1(a, b, & c) + ≥3 in B + ≥1 in C
or
A2 + ≥4 in B + ≥1 in C,
then criteria met
MAN < >

If A1(a, b, & c) + ≥3 in B +
none in C
or
A2 + ≥4 in B + none in C,
then criteria met
HYPOMAN < >

Duration

1. ______________ (years old)
2. < > ____________ (years old)
3. MAN < > ________ (weeks)
   HYPO < > _______ (days)

*DUR met for MAN < >
*DUR met for HYPOMAN < >

Impairment

1. < > home
2. < > school
3. < > peers

ENU

1. < >
2. <a> <b>
3. <a> <b>

Criteria

If 1, ≥1 in 2, 3a, and 3b, then criteria met

ENU < >

Duration

1. ________ (years old)
2. < > ________ (years old)
3. <a> ________ (x/week)
   <b> ________ (months)

*DUR met for ENU < >

Impairment

1. < > home
2. < > school
3. < > peers

Type

Nocturnal < >
Diurnal < >
Both < >

ENC

1. < >
2. < >

Criteria

If both 1 & 2, then criteria met

ENC < >

Duration

1. ________ (years old)
2. < > ________ (years old)
3. <a> ________ (x/month)
   <b> ________ (months)

*DUR met for ENC < >

Impairment

1. < > home
2. < > school
3. < > peers

SCZ/PSY

A. Psychotic Symptoms
1. <a> <b> <c> <d> <e>
2. <a> <b> <c> <d> <e> <f>
3. < >
4. < >
5. < >

B. Interference
1. < >
2. < >
3. < >

Criteria

If ≥2 in A and ≥1 in B, then criteria met

SCZ < >

If ≥1 in A, then criteria met

PSY < >

Duration

1. ________ (years old)
2. < > ________ (years old)
3. < > ________ (months)

*DUR met for SCZ < >

*DUR met for PSY < >

Impairment

1. < > home
2. < > school
3. < > peers

STRESSORS

A. Child Abuse/Neglect
1. <a> <b> <c>
2. <a> <b> <c> <d>
3. <a> <b> <c> <d>
4. < >
5. < >

Duration

1. ________
2. < > ________
3. ________
4. ________
5. < >

B. Other Stressors
1. <a> <b> <c> <d> <e>
2. < >
3. <a> <b>
4. <a> <b> <c>
5. <a> <b>
6. <a> <b>
7. <a> ________
   <b>
8. <a> <b> <c> <d>
9. < > ________
   ____
   ____
10. < >
11. < > ________
   ____
   ____

P-ChIPS Scoring Form
Profile Sheet

Child's Number: ______________________ Date: ______________
Child's Name: ______________________ Time Started: ______________
Date of Birth: ______________ Age: ______________ Time Ended: ______________
Race: ______________ Sex: ______________ Interviewer: ______________
Informant's Name: ______________________
Informant's Relationship (circle one): Mother, Father, Stepmother, Stepfather, Guardian, Other: ______________

	Disorder	Symptoms	Diagnosis	Duration	Clinician's Diagnosis
ADHD	**Attention-Deficit/Hyperactivity Disorder** *Type:* Inattentive, Hyperactive–Impulsive, Combined	<>	<>	<>	**Axis I**
ODD	**Oppositional Defiant Disorder**	<>	<>	<>	
CD	**Conduct Disorder** *Onset:* Childhood, Adolescent *Severity:* Mild, Moderate, Severe	<>	<>	<>	
SUBAB	**Substance Abuse** *Substance(s):* ____________	<>	<>	<>	
PHO	**Specific Phobia** *Type:* ____________	<>	<>	<>	**Axis II**
SOCPHO	**Social Phobia**	<>	<>	<>	
SEPANX	**Separation Anxiety Disorder**	<>	<>	<>	**Axis III**
GENANX	**General Anxiety Disorder**	<>	<>	<>	
OCD	**Obsessive-Compulsive Disorder**	<>	<>	<>	
PTSD	**Posttraumatic Stress Disorder** *Type:* Acute, Chronic *Onset:* Regular, Delayed	<>	<>	<>	**Axis IV**
ASD	**Acute Stress Disorder**	<>	<>	<>	
ANO	**Anorexia**	<>	<>	<>	**Axis V**
BUL	**Bulimia**	<>	<>	<>	**current:**
DEP	**Major Depressive Disorder**	<>	<>	<>	**past year:**
DYS	**Dysthymic Disorder**	<>	<>	<>	
MAN	**Mania**	<>	<>	<>	
HYPOMAN	**Hypomania**	<>	<>	<>	
ENU	**Enuresis** *Type:* Nocturnal, Diurnal, Both	<>	<>	<>	
ENC	**Encopresis**	<>	<>	<>	
SCZ	**Schizophrenia**	<>	<>	<>	
PSY	**Psychosis**	<>	<>	<>	

Psychosocial Stressors:

Other Stressors:

Behavioral Observations

Appearance:

Affect:

Effort:

Level of Activity:

Unusual Behaviors:

Presenting Problem

Home
1.
2.

School
1.
2.
3.
4.
5.

Peers/Work
1.
2.
3.
4.
5.

Medication
Type:
Dosage:

Child's Name: ____________________

Date: ____________

ADHD	ODD	CD
A. Inattention 1. <a> <b> 2. < > 3. <a> <b> 4. <a> <b> <c> 5. < > 6. < > 7. < > 8. <a> <b> 9. <a> <b> B. Hyperactivity–Impulsivity 1. <a> <b> 2. <a> <b> 3. < > 4. <a> <b> 5. < > 6. <a> <b> 7. < > 8. <a> <b> 9. <a> <b> <c>	1. <a> <b> 2. <a> <b> 3. <a> <b> <c> <d> 4. < > 5. <a> <b> 6. < > 7. < > 8. < >	1. < > 2. <a> <b> 3. < > 4. < > 5. < > 6. < > 7. <a> <b> 8. <a> <b> 9. < > 10. <a> <b> 11. < > 12. < > 13. < > 14. < > 15. <a> <b>
Criteria If ≥6 in *A only*, then criteria met Inattentive < > If ≥6 in *B only*, then criteria met Hyperactive–Impulsive < > If ≥6 in A *and* ≥6 in B, then criteria met Combined < >	**Criteria** If ≥4, then criteria met ODD < >	**Criteria** If ≥3, then criteria met CD < >
Duration 1. ____________ (years old) 2. < > __________ (years old) 3. < > __________ (months) * DUR met for ADHD < >	**Duration** 1. ____________ (years old) 2. < > __________ (years old) 3. < > __________ (months) * DUR met for ODD < >	**Duration** 1. ____________ (years old) 2. < > __________ (years old) 3. < > __________ (months) * DUR met for CD < >
Impairment 1. < > home 2. < > school 3. < > peers	**Impairment** 1. < > home 2. < > school 3. < > peers	**Impairment** 1. < > home 2. < > school 3. < > peers
		Type Childhood Onset < > Adolescent Onset < > Mild < > Moderate < > Severe < >

SUB AB

1. < >
   <a>____________________
   <b>____________________
   <c>____________________
   ____
2. < > ____________________
3. < > ____________________
4. < > ____________________

Duration
1. ____________ (years old)
2. < > _________ (years old)
   _________ (months)

* DUR met for SUB AB < >

Impairment
1. <a> <b>
2. < >
3. <a> <b>
4. < >

Criteria
If any use (Q1–4) and any impairment (1–4), then criteria met SUB AB < >

Type(s) ____________________
____
____
____

PHO

1. ________________________
   ____
   ____
2. <a> <b>
3. <a> <b>
4. <ai> <aii> <aiii> <aiv> <b>
5. <a> <b>

Criteria
If 1–4, then criteria met PHO < >

Duration
1. ____________ (years old)
2. < > _________ (years old)
3. < > _________ (months)

* DUR met for PHO < >

Impairment
1. < > home
2. < > school
3. < > peers

Type(s)

Animal	< >
Natural Environment	< >
Blood–Injection–Injury	< >
Situational	< >
Other ________________	< >

SOCIAL PHO

1. <a> <b>
2. < >
3. <a> <b>
4. <ai> <aii> <aiii> <aiv> <b>
5. < >

Criteria
If 1–4, then criteria met SOCIAL PHO < >

Duration
1. ____________ (years old)
2. < > _________ (years old)
3. < > _________ (months)

*DUR met for SOCIAL PHO < >

Impairment
1. < > home
2. < > school
3. < > peers

SEP ANX	GEN ANX	OCD
1. <a> <b> 2. <a> <b> 3. < > 4. <a> <b> 5. <a> <b> 6. <a> <b> 7. <a> <b> 8. <a> <b>	1. < > ____________ ____________ ____________ ____________ ____________ 2. <a> <b> 3. <a> <b> <c> <d> <e> <f>	A. Compulsions 1. < > ____________ 2. <a> ____________ <b> 3. < > B. Obsessions 1. <a> ____________ <b> ____________ <c> ____________ 2. <a> <b> <c> 3. < > C. Interference 1. <a> <b> <c>
Criteria If $\geq$3, then criteria met SEP ANX < >	**Criteria** If 1–3, then criteria met GEN ANX < >	**Criteria** If A1, A2, & C, then criteria met Compulsions < > If B1, B2, & C, then criteria met Obsessions < > If Compulsions + and/or Obsessions +, then criteria met OCD < >
Duration 1. ____________ (years old) 2. < > __________ (years old) 3. < > __________ (weeks) *DUR met for SEP ANX < >	**Duration** 1. ____________ (years old) 2. < > __________ (years old) 3. < > __________ (months) *DUR met for GEN ANX < >	**Duration** 1. ____________ (years old) 2. < > __________ (years old) __________ (months) *DUR met for OCD < >
Impairment 1. < > home 2. < > school 3. < > peers	**Impairment** 1. < > home 2. < > school 3. < > peers	**Impairment** 1. < > home 2. < > school 3. < > peers

STRESS (ASD/PTSD)	ANO	BUL
A. Exposure 1. <a> <b> ____________ 2. <a> <b> <c> <d> <e> 3. < > ____________ B. Dissociation 1. <a> <b> <c> <d> 2. < > 3. < > 4. < > 5. < > C. Reexperiencing 1. <a> <b> <c> 2. <a> <b> 3. <a> <b> 4. <a> <b> 5. < > D. Avoidance 1. <a> <b> 2. <a> <b> <c> 3. < > 4. <a> <b> 5. <a> <b> 6. <a> <b> 7. <a> <b> E. Hyperarousal 1. <a> <b> 2. <a> <b> 3. < > 4. < > 5. < >	1. <a> <b> 2. <a> ht: ____________ wt: ____________ <b> ht: ____________ wt: ____________ 3. <a> <b> <c> 4. <a> <b> <c> 5. < >	1. < > ____________ ____________ 2. <a> <b> <c> <d> 3. <a> <b> <c> <d> 4. <a> <b>
Criteria If A1 & A2, ≥3 in B, ≥1 in C, ≥3 in D, and ≥2 in E, then criteria met ASD < > If A1 & A2, ≥1 in C, ≥3 in D, and ≥2 in E, then criteria met PTSD < >	**Criteria** If 1–4 (&5 for pubescent girls), then criteria met ANO < >	**Criteria** If 1–4, then criteria met BUL < >
Duration 1. ____________ (years old) 2. < > __________ (years old) 3. a. < > ________ (weeks) b. < > c. < > ________ (days) 4. < > __________ (months) *DUR met for ASD < > *DUR met for PTSD < >	**Duration** 1. __________ (years old) 2. < > ________ (years old) 3. < > ________ (months) *DUR met for ANO < >	**Duration** 1. __________ (years old) 2. < > ________ (years old) 3. a. < > _____ (#/week) b. < > _____ (months) *DUR met for BUL < >
Impairment 1. < > home 2. < > school 3. < > peers **Type (PTSD)** Acute < > Regular Onset < > Chronic < > Delayed Onset < >	**Impairment** 1. < > home 2. < > school 3. < > peers	**Impairment** 1. < > home 2. < > school 3. < > peers

DEP/DYS (MDD/DD)

A. Dysphoric Mood
1. <a> <b> <c>
2. <a> <bi> <bii> <biii> <c> <d>

B. Loss of Interest
1. <a> <b>
2. <a> <b> <c>

C. Appetite Changes
1. <a> <b> <c>
2. <a> <b>

D. Sleep Changes
Bedtime: __________
Wakeup: __________
1. <a> <b> <c>
2. <a> <b>

E. Psychomotor Changes
1. <a> <b> <c> <d>
2. <a> <b>

F. Low Energy
1. <a> <b> <c> <d>

G. Guilt
1. <a> <b> <c> <d>
2. <a> <b>

H. Impaired Concentration
1. <a> <b> <c> <d> <e>
2. < >

I. Hopelessness
1. <a> <b> <c>

J. Morbid/Suicidal Thoughts
1. <a> <b>
2. <a> <b> <c> <d> <e>

____
____
____
____
____

DEP/DYS (MDD/DD)

Criteria

If A &/or B & ≥5 of A–H or J, then criteria met
MDD < >

If A & ≥2 of C, D, F, G, H, or I, then criteria met
DD < >

Duration

1. ______________ (years old)
2. < > ______________ (years old)
3. MDD < > ________ (weeks)
   DD < > ________ (months)

*DUR met for MDD < >
*DUR met for DD < >

Impairment

1. < > home
2. < > school
3. < > peers

MAN/HYPOMAN

A. Elevated Mood
1. <a> ______________________
   <b> ______________________
   <c> ______________________
2. < > ______________________

B. Other Symptoms
1. <a> ______________________
   <b>
2. <a> <b> <c> __________
3. <a> <b> <c> <d>
4. <a> <b> <c>
5. < >
6. <a> <b> <c> <d> <e>
7. <a> <b> <c> <d>

C. Interference
1. < >
2. < >

Criteria

If A1(a, b, & c) + ≥3 in B + ≥1 in C
or
A2 + ≥4 in B + ≥1 in C, then criteria met
MAN < >

If A1(a, b, & c) + ≥3 in B + none in C
or
A2 + ≥4 in B + none in C, then criteria met
HYPOMAN < >

Duration

1. ______________ (years old)
2. < > ______________ (years old)
3. MAN < > ________ (weeks)
   HYPO < > ________ (days)

*DUR met for MAN < >
*DUR met for HYPOMAN < >

Impairment

1. < > home
2. < > school
3. < > peers

ENU

1. < >
2. <a> <b>
3. <a> <b>

Criteria

If 1, ≥1 in 2, 3a, and 3b, then criteria met

ENU < >

Duration

1. ______ (years old)
2. < > ______ (years old)
3. <a> ______ (x/week)
   <b> ______ (months)

*DUR met for ENU < >

Impairment

1. < > home
2. < > school
3. < > peers

Type

Nocturnal < >
Diurnal < >
Both < >

ENC

1. < >
2. < >

Criteria

If both 1 & 2, then criteria met

ENC < >

Duration

1. ______ (years old)
2. < > ______ (years old)
3. <a> ______ (x/month)
   <b> ______ (months)

*DUR met for ENC < >

Impairment

1. < > home
2. < > school
3. < > peers

SCZ/PSY

A. Psychotic Symptoms
1. <a> <b> <c> <d> <e>
2. <a> <b> <c> <d> <e> <f>
3. < >
4. < >
5. < >

B. Interference
1. < >
2. < >
3. < >

Criteria

If ≥2 in A and ≥1 in B, then criteria met

SCZ < >

If ≥1 in A, then criteria met

PSY < >

Duration

1. ______ (years old)
2. < > ______ (years old)
3. < > ______ (months)

*DUR met for SCZ < >
*DUR met for PSY < >

Impairment

1. < > home
2. < > school
3. < > peers

STRESSORS

A. Child Abuse/Neglect
1. <a> <b> <c>
2. <a> <b> <c> <d>
3. <a> <b> <c> <d>
4. < >
5. < >

Duration

1. ______
2. < > ______
3. ______
4. ______
5. < >

B. Other Stressors
1. <a> <b> <c> <d> <e>
2. < >
3. <a> <b>
4. <a> <b> <c>
5. <a> <b>
6. <a> <b>
7. <a> ______
   <b>
8. <a> <b> <c> <d>
9. < > ______
   ______
   ______
10. < >
11. < > ______
    ______
    ______

P-ChIPS Scoring Form
Profile Sheet

Child's Number: ______________________________ Date: ______________

Child's Name: ______________________________ Time Started: ______________

Date of Birth: ______________ Age: ______________ Time Ended: ______________

Race: ______________ Sex: ______________ Interviewer: ______________

Informant's Name: ______________________________

Informant's Relationship (circle one): Mother, Father, Stepmother, Stepfather, Guardian, Other: ______________

	Disorder	Symptoms	Diagnosis	Duration	Clinician's Diagnosis
ADHD	**Attention-Deficit/Hyperactivity Disorder**	<>	<>	<>	**Axis I**
	Type: Inattentive, Hyperactive–Impulsive, Combined				
ODD	**Oppositional Defiant Disorder**	<>	<>	<>	
CD	**Conduct Disorder**	<>	<>	<>	
	Onset: Childhood, Adolescent				
	Severity: Mild, Moderate, Severe				
SUBAB	**Substance Abuse**	<>	<>	<>	
	Substance(s): ______________				
PHO	**Specific Phobia**	<>	<>	<>	**Axis II**
	Type: ______________				
SOCPHO	**Social Phobia**	<>	<>	<>	
SEPANX	**Separation Anxiety Disorder**	<>	<>	<>	**Axis III**
GENANX	**General Anxiety Disorder**	<>	<>	<>	
OCD	**Obsessive-Compulsive Disorder**	<>	<>	<>	
PTSD	**Posttraumatic Stress Disorder**	<>	<>	<>	**Axis IV**
	Type: Acute, Chronic				
	Onset: Regular, Delayed				
ASD	**Acute Stress Disorder**	<>	<>	<>	
ANO	**Anorexia**	<>	<>	<>	**Axis V**
BUL	**Bulimia**	<>	<>	<>	**current:**
DEP	**Major Depressive Disorder**	<>	<>	<>	**past year:**
DYS	**Dysthymic Disorder**	<>	<>	<>	
MAN	**Mania**	<>	<>	<>	
HYPOMAN	**Hypomania**	<>	<>	<>	
ENU	**Enuresis**	<>	<>	<>	
	Type: Nocturnal, Diurnal, Both				
ENC	**Encopresis**	<>	<>	<>	
SCZ	**Schizophrenia**	<>	<>	<>	
PSY	**Psychosis**	<>	<>	<>	

Psychosocial Stressors:

Other Stressors:

Behavioral Observations

Appearance:

Affect:

Effort:

Level of Activity:

Unusual Behaviors:

Presenting Problem

Home

1.

2.

School

1.

2.

3.

4.

5.

Peers/Work

1.

2.

3.

4.

5.

Medication

Type:

Dosage:

Child's Name: ______________________________

Date: ________________

ADHD	ODD	CD
A. Inattention 1. <a> <b> 2. < > 3. <a> <b> 4. <a> <b> <c> 5. < > 6. < > 7. < > 8. <a> <b> 9. <a> <b> B. Hyperactivity–Impulsivity 1. <a> <b> 2. <a> <b> 3. < > 4. <a> <b> 5. < > 6. <a> <b> 7. < > 8. <a> <b> 9. <a> <b> <c>	1. <a> <b> 2. <a> <b> 3. <a> <b> <c> <d> 4. < > 5. <a> <b> 6. < > 7. < > 8. < >	1. < > 2. <a> <b> 3. < > 4. < > 5. < > 6. < > 7. <a> <b> 8. <a> <b> 9. < > 10. <a> <b> 11. < > 12. < > 13. < > 14. < > 15. <a> <b>
Criteria If ≥6 in *A only*, then criteria met Inattentive < > If ≥6 in *B only*, then criteria met Hyperactive–Impulsive < > If ≥6 in A *and* ≥6 in B, then criteria met Combined < >	**Criteria** If ≥4, then criteria met ODD < >	**Criteria** If ≥3, then criteria met CD < >
Duration 1. __________ (years old) 2. < > ________ (years old) 3. < > ________ (months) * DUR met for ADHD < >	**Duration** 1. __________ (years old) 2. < > ________ (years old) 3. < > ________ (months) * DUR met for ODD < >	**Duration** 1. __________ (years old) 2. < > ________ (years old) 3. < > ________ (months) * DUR met for CD < >
Impairment 1. < > home 2. < > school 3. < > peers	**Impairment** 1. < > home 2. < > school 3. < > peers	**Impairment** 1. < > home 2. < > school 3. < > peers
		Type Childhood Onset < > Adolescent Onset < > Mild < > Moderate < > Severe < >

SUB AB

1. < >
   <a>______________________
   <b>______________________
   <c>______________________
   ____
2. < > ______________________
3. < > ______________________
4. < > ______________________

Duration

1. ____________ (years old)
2. < > __________ (years old)
   __________ (months)

* DUR met for SUB AB < >

Impairment

1. <a> <b>
2. < >
3. <a> <b>
4. < >

Criteria

If any use (Q1–4) and any impairment (1–4), then criteria met SUB AB < >

Type(s) ______________________
____
____
____

PHO

1. ______________________
   ____
   ____
2. <a> <b>
3. <a> <b>
4. <ai> <aii> <aiii> <aiv> <b>
5. <a> <b>

Criteria

If 1–4, then criteria met PHO < >

Duration

1. ____________ (years old)
2. < > __________ (years old)
3. < > __________ (months)

* DUR met for PHO < >

Impairment

1. < > home
2. < > school
3. < > peers

Type(s)

Animal	< >
Natural Environment	< >
Blood–Injection–Injury	< >
Situational	< >
Other ________________	< >

SOCIAL PHO

1. <a> <b>
2. < >
3. <a> <b>
4. <ai> <aii> <aiii> <aiv> <b>
5. < >

Criteria

If 1–4, then criteria met SOCIAL PHO < >

Duration

1. ____________ (years old)
2. < > __________ (years old)
3. < > __________ (months)

*DUR met for SOCIAL PHO < >

Impairment

1. < > home
2. < > school
3. < > peers

SEP ANX	GEN ANX	OCD
1. <a> <b> 2. <a> <b> 3. < > 4. <a> <b> 5. <a> <b> 6. <a> <b> 7. <a> <b> 8. <a> <b>	1. < > ____________ ____________ ____________ ____________ ____________ 2. <a> <b> 3. <a> <b> <c> <d> <e> <f>	A. Compulsions 1. < > ____________ 2. <a> ____________ <b> 3. < > B. Obsessions 1. <a> ____________ <b> ____________ <c> ____________ 2. <a> <b> <c> 3. < > C. Interference 1. <a> <b> <c>
Criteria If ≥3, then criteria met SEP ANX < >	**Criteria** If 1–3, then criteria met GEN ANX < >	**Criteria** If A1, A2, & C, then criteria met Compulsions < > If B1, B2, & C, then criteria met Obsessions < > If Compulsions + and/or Obsessions +, then criteria met OCD < >
Duration 1. ____________ (years old) 2. < > ____________ (years old) 3. < > ____________ (weeks) *DUR met for SEP ANX < >	**Duration** 1. ____________ (years old) 2. < > ____________ (years old) 3. < > ____________ (months) *DUR met for GEN ANX < >	**Duration** 1. ____________ (years old) 2. < > ____________ (years old) ____________ (months) *DUR met for OCD < >
Impairment 1. < > home 2. < > school 3. < > peers	**Impairment** 1. < > home 2. < > school 3. < > peers	**Impairment** 1. < > home 2. < > school 3. < > peers

STRESS (ASD/PTSD)	**ANO**	**BUL**
A. Exposure 1. <a> <b> ______________ 2. <a> <b> <c> <d> <e> 3. < > ______________ B. Dissociation 1. <a> <b> <c> <d> 2. < > 3. < > 4. < > 5. < > C. Reexperiencing 1. <a> <b> <c> 2. <a> <b> 3. <a> <b> 4. <a> <b> 5. < > D. Avoidance 1. <a> <b> 2. <a> <b> <c> 3. < > 4. <a> <b> 5. <a> <b> 6. <a> <b> 7. <a> <b> E. Hyperarousal 1. <a> <b> 2. <a> <b> 3. < > 4. < > 5. < >	1. <a> <b> 2. <a> ht: ____________ wt: ____________ <b> ht: ____________ wt: ____________ 3. <a> <b> <c> 4. <a> <b> <c> 5. < >	1. < > ______________ ______________ 2. <a> <b> <c> <d> 3. <a> <b> <c> <d> 4. <a> <b>
Criteria If A1 & A2, $\geq$3 in B, $\geq$1 in C, $\geq$3 in D, and $\geq$2 in E, then criteria met ASD < > If A1 & A2, $\geq$1 in C, $\geq$3 in D, and $\geq$2 in E, then criteria met PTSD < >	**Criteria** If 1–4 (&5 for pubescent girls), then criteria met ANO < >	**Criteria** If 1–4, then criteria met BUL < >
Duration 1. ____________ (years old) 2. < > ________ (years old) 3. a. < > ______ (weeks) b. < > c. < > ______ (days) 4. < > __________ (months) *DUR met for ASD < > *DUR met for PTSD < >	**Duration** 1. __________ (years old) 2. < > ______ (years old) 3. < > ______ (months) *DUR met for ANO < >	**Duration** 1. __________ (years old) 2. < > ______ (years old) 3. a. < > _____ (#/week) b. < > _____ (months) *DUR met for BUL < >
Impairment 1. < > home 2. < > school 3. < > peers **Type (PTSD)** Acute < > Regular Onset < > Chronic < > Delayed Onset < >	**Impairment** 1. < > home 2. < > school 3. < > peers	**Impairment** 1. < > home 2. < > school 3. < > peers

DEP/DYS (MDD/DD)

A. Dysphoric Mood
  1. <a> <b> <c>
  2. <a> <bi> <bii> <biii> <c> <d>

B. Loss of Interest
  1. <a> <b>
  2. <a> <b> <c>

C. Appetite Changes
  1. <a> <b> <c>
  2. <a> <b>

D. Sleep Changes
  Bedtime: ______
  Wakeup: ______
  1. <a> <b> <c>
  2. <a> <b>

E. Psychomotor Changes
  1. <a> <b> <c> <d>
  2. <a> <b>

F. Low Energy
  1. <a> <b> <c> <d>

G. Guilt
  1. <a> <b> <c> <d>
  2. <a> <b>

H. Impaired Concentration
  1. <a> <b> <c> <d> <e>
  2. < >

I. Hopelessness
  1. <a> <b> <c>

J. Morbid/Suicidal Thoughts
  1. <a> <b>
  2. <a> <b> <c> <d> <e>

______
______
______
______
______

DEP/DYS (MDD/DD)

Criteria

If A &/or B & ≥5 of A–H or J,
then criteria met
MDD < >

If A & ≥2 of C, D, F, G, H, or I,
then criteria met
DD < >

Duration

1. ______ (years old)
2. < > ______ (years old)
3. MDD < > ______ (weeks)
   DD < > ______ (months)

*DUR met for MDD < >
*DUR met for DD < >

Impairment

1. < > home
2. < > school
3. < > peers

MAN/HYPOMAN

A. Elevated Mood
  1. <a> ______
     <b> ______
     <c> ______
  2. < > ______

B. Other Symptoms
  1. <a> ______
     <b>
  2. <a> <b> <c> ______
  3. <a> <b> <c> <d>
  4. <a> <b> <c>
  5. < >
  6. <a> <b> <c> <d> <e>
  7. <a> <b> <c> <d>

C. Interference
  1. < >
  2. < >

Criteria

If A1(a, b, & c) + ≥3 in B + ≥1 in C
or
A2 + ≥4 in B + ≥1 in C,
then criteria met
MAN < >

If A1(a, b, & c) + ≥3 in B +
none in C
or
A2 + ≥4 in B + none in C,
then criteria met
HYPOMAN < >

Duration

1. ______ (years old)
2. < > ______ (years old)
3. MAN < > ______ (weeks)
   HYPO < > ______ (days)

*DUR met for MAN < >
*DUR met for HYPOMAN < >

Impairment

1. < > home
2. < > school
3. < > peers

ENU

1. < >
2. <a> <b>
3. <a> <b>

Criteria

If 1, ≥1 in 2, 3a, and 3b,
then criteria met
ENU < >

Duration

1. ______________ (years old)
2. < > __________ (years old)
3. <a> __________ (x/week)
   <b> __________ (months)

*DUR met for ENU < >

Impairment

1. < > home
2. < > school
3. < > peers

Type

Nocturnal	< >
Diurnal	< >
Both	< >

ENC

1. < >
2. < >

Criteria

If both 1 & 2, then criteria met
ENC < >

Duration

1. ______________ (years old)
2. < > __________ (years old)
3. <a> __________ (x/month)
   <b> __________ (months)

*DUR met for ENC < >

Impairment

1. < > home
2. < > school
3. < > peers

SCZ/PSY

A. Psychotic Symptoms
1. <a> <b> <c> <d> <e>
2. <a> <b> <c> <d> <e> <f>
3. < >
4. < >
5. < >

B. Interference
1. < >
2. < >
3. < >

Criteria

If ≥2 in A and ≥1 in B,
then criteria met
SCZ < >

If ≥1 in A, then criteria met
PSY < >

Duration

1. ______________ (years old)
2. < > __________ (years old)
3. < > __________ (months)

*DUR met for SCZ < >
*DUR met for PSY < >

Impairment

1. < > home
2. < > school
3. < > peers

STRESSORS

A. Child Abuse/Neglect
1. <a> <b> <c>
2. <a> <b> <c> <d>
3. <a> <b> <c> <d>
4. < >
5. < >

Duration

1. ______________
2. < > ______________
3. ______________
4. ______________
5. < >

B. Other Stressors
1. <a> <b> <c> <d> <e>
2. < >
3. <a> <b>
4. <a> <b> <c>
5. <a> <b>
6. <a> <b>
7. <a> ______________
   <b>
8. <a> <b> <c> <d>
9. < > ______________
   ____
   ____
10. < >
11. < > ______________
   ____
   ____

P-ChIPS Scoring Form
Profile Sheet

Child's Number: ______________________ Date: ______________

Child's Name: ______________________ Time Started: ______________

Date of Birth: ______________ Age: ______________ Time Ended: ______________

Race: ______________ Sex: ______________ Interviewer: ______________

Informant's Name: ______________________

Informant's Relationship (circle one): Mother, Father, Stepmother, Stepfather, Guardian, Other: ______________

	Disorder	Symptoms	Diagnosis	Duration	Clinician's Diagnosis
ADHD	**Attention-Deficit/Hyperactivity Disorder**	<>	<>	<>	**Axis I**
	Type: Inattentive, Hyperactive–Impulsive, Combined				
ODD	**Oppositional Defiant Disorder**	<>	<>	<>	
CD	**Conduct Disorder**	<>	<>	<>	
	Onset: Childhood, Adolescent				
	Severity: Mild, Moderate, Severe				
SUBAB	**Substance Abuse**	<>	<>	<>	
	Substance(s): ______________				
PHO	**Specific Phobia**	<>	<>	<>	**Axis II**
	Type: ______________				
SOCPHO	**Social Phobia**	<>	<>	<>	
SEPANX	**Separation Anxiety Disorder**	<>	<>	<>	**Axis III**
GENANX	**General Anxiety Disorder**	<>	<>	<>	
OCD	**Obsessive-Compulsive Disorder**	<>	<>	<>	
PTSD	**Posttraumatic Stress Disorder**	<>	<>	<>	**Axis IV**
	Type: Acute, Chronic				
	Onset: Regular, Delayed				
ASD	**Acute Stress Disorder**	<>	<>	<>	
ANO	**Anorexia**	<>	<>	<>	**Axis V**
BUL	**Bulimia**	<>	<>	<>	**current:**
DEP	**Major Depressive Disorder**	<>	<>	<>	**past year:**
DYS	**Dysthymic Disorder**	<>	<>	<>	
MAN	**Mania**	<>	<>	<>	
HYPOMAN	**Hypomania**	<>	<>	<>	
ENU	**Enuresis**	<>	<>	<>	
	Type: Nocturnal, Diurnal, Both				
ENC	**Encopresis**	<>	<>	<>	
SCZ	**Schizophrenia**	<>	<>	<>	
PSY	**Psychosis**	<>	<>	<>	

Psychosocial Stressors:

Other Stressors:

Behavioral Observations

Appearance:

Affect:

Effort:

Level of Activity:

Unusual Behaviors:

Presenting Problem

Home

1.

2.

School

1.

2.

3.

4.

5.

Peers/Work

1.

2.

3.

4.

5.

Medication

Type:

Dosage:

Child's Name: ______________________________

Date: ______________

ADHD	ODD	CD
A. Inattention 1. <a> <b> 2. < > 3. <a> <b> 4. <a> <b> <c> 5. < > 6. < > 7. < > 8. <a> <b> 9. <a> <b> B. Hyperactivity–Impulsivity 1. <a> <b> 2. <a> <b> 3. < > 4. <a> <b> 5. < > 6. <a> <b> 7. < > 8. <a> <b> 9. <a> <b> <c>	1. <a> <b> 2. <a> <b> 3. <a> <b> <c> <d> 4. < > 5. <a> <b> 6. < > 7. < > 8. < >	1. < > 2. <a> <b> 3. < > 4. < > 5. < > 6. < > 7. <a> <b> 8. <a> <b> 9. < > 10. <a> <b> 11. < > 12. < > 13. < > 14. < > 15. <a> <b>
Criteria If ≥6 in *A only*, then criteria met Inattentive < > If ≥6 in *B only*, then criteria met Hyperactive–Impulsive < > If ≥6 in A *and* ≥6 in B, then criteria met Combined < >	**Criteria** If ≥4, then criteria met ODD < >	**Criteria** If ≥3, then criteria met CD < >
Duration 1. ____________ (years old) 2. < > _________ (years old) 3. < > __________ (months) * DUR met for ADHD < >	**Duration** 1. ____________ (years old) 2. < > _________ (years old) 3. < > __________ (months) * DUR met for ODD < >	**Duration** 1. ____________ (years old) 2. < > _________ (years old) 3. < > __________ (months) * DUR met for CD < >
Impairment 1. < > home 2. < > school 3. < > peers	**Impairment** 1. < > home 2. < > school 3. < > peers	**Impairment** 1. < > home 2. < > school 3. < > peers **Type** Childhood Onset < > Adolescent Onset < > Mild < > Moderate < > Severe < >

SUB AB

1. < >
   <a>______________________
   <b>______________________
   <c>______________________
   ____
2. < > ______________________
3. < > ______________________
4. < > ______________________

Duration

1. ____________ (years old)
2. < > __________ (years old)
   __________ (months)

* DUR met for SUB AB < >

Impairment

1. <a> <b>
2. < >
3. <a> <b>
4. < >

Criteria

If any use (Q1–4) and any impairment (1–4), then criteria met SUB AB < >

Type(s) ____________________

____
____
____

PHO

1. ________________________
   ____
   ____
2. <a> <b>
3. <a> <b>
4. <ai> <aii> <aiii> <aiv> <b>
5. <a> <b>

Criteria

If 1–4, then criteria met PHO < >

Duration

1. ____________ (years old)
2. < > __________ (years old)
3. < > __________ (months)

* DUR met for PHO < >

Impairment

1. < > home
2. < > school
3. < > peers

Type(s)

Animal	< >
Natural Environment	< >
Blood–Injection–Injury	< >
Situational	< >
Other ________________	< >

SOCIAL PHO

1. <a> <b>
2. < >
3. <a> <b>
4. <ai> <aii> <aiii> <aiv> <b>
5. < >

Criteria

If 1–4, then criteria met SOCIAL PHO < >

Duration

1. ____________ (years old)
2. < > __________ (years old)
3. < > __________ (months)

*DUR met for SOCIAL PHO < >

Impairment

1. < > home
2. < > school
3. < > peers

SEP ANX	**GEN ANX**	**OCD**
1. <a> <b> 2. <a> <b> 3. < > 4. <a> <b> 5. <a> <b> 6. <a> <b> 7. <a> <b> 8. <a> <b>	1. < > ____________ ____________ ____________ ____________ ____________ 2. <a> <b> 3. <a> <b> <c> <d> <e> <f>	A. Compulsions 1. < > ____________ 2. <a> ____________ <b> 3. < > B. Obsessions 1. <a> ____________ <b> ____________ <c> ____________ 2. <a> <b> <c> 3. < > C. Interference 1. <a> <b> <c>
Criteria If ≥3, then criteria met SEP ANX < >	**Criteria** If 1–3, then criteria met GEN ANX < >	**Criteria** If A1, A2, & C, then criteria met Compulsions < > If B1, B2, & C, then criteria met Obsessions < > If Compulsions + and/or Obsessions +, then criteria met OCD < >
Duration 1. ____________ (years old) 2. < > __________ (years old) 3. < > __________ (weeks) *DUR met for SEP ANX < >	**Duration** 1. ____________ (years old) 2. < > __________ (years old) 3. < > __________ (months) *DUR met for GEN ANX < >	**Duration** 1. ____________ (years old) 2. < > __________ (years old) __________ (months) *DUR met for OCD < >
Impairment 1. < > home 2. < > school 3. < > peers	**Impairment** 1. < > home 2. < > school 3. < > peers	**Impairment** 1. < > home 2. < > school 3. < > peers

STRESS (ASD/PTSD)	ANO	BUL
A. Exposure 1. <a> <b> ____________ 2. <a> <b> <c> <d> <e> 3. < > ____________ B. Dissociation 1. <a> <b> <c> <d> 2. < > 3. < > 4. < > 5. < > C. Reexperiencing 1. <a> <b> <c> 2. <a> <b> 3. <a> <b> 4. <a> <b> 5. < > D. Avoidance 1. <a> <b> 2. <a> <b> <c> 3. < > 4. <a> <b> 5. <a> <b> 6. <a> <b> 7. <a> <b> E. Hyperarousal 1. <a> <b> 2. <a> <b> 3. < > 4. < > 5. < >	1. <a> <b> 2. <a> ht: ________ wt: ________ <b> ht: ________ wt: ________ 3. <a> <b> <c> 4. <a> <b> <c> 5. < >	1. < > ____________ ____________ 2. <a> <b> <c> <d> 3. <a> <b> <c> <d> 4. <a> <b>
Criteria If A1 & A2, $\geq$3 in B, $\geq$1 in C, $\geq$3 in D, and $\geq$2 in E, then criteria met ASD < > If A1 & A2, $\geq$1 in C, $\geq$3 in D, and $\geq$2 in E, then criteria met PTSD < >	**Criteria** If 1–4 (&5 for pubescent girls), then criteria met ANO < >	**Criteria** If 1–4, then criteria met BUL < >
Duration 1. ________ (years old) 2. < > ________ (years old) 3. a. < > ______ (weeks) b. < > c. < > ______ (days) 4. < > ________ (months) *DUR met for ASD < > *DUR met for PTSD < >	**Duration** 1. ________ (years old) 2. < > ______ (years old) 3. < > ______ (months) *DUR met for ANO < >	**Duration** 1. ________ (years old) 2. < > ______ (years old) 3. a. < > _____ (#/week) b. < > _____ (months) *DUR met for BUL < >
Impairment 1. < > home 2. < > school 3. < > peers **Type (PTSD)** Acute < > Regular Onset < > Chronic < > Delayed Onset < >	**Impairment** 1. < > home 2. < > school 3. < > peers	**Impairment** 1. < > home 2. < > school 3. < > peers

DEP/DYS (MDD/DD)

A. Dysphoric Mood
   1. <a> <b> <c>
   2. <a> <bi> <bii> <biii> <c> <d>

B. Loss of Interest
   1. <a> <b>
   2. <a> <b> <c>

C. Appetite Changes
   1. <a> <b> <c>
   2. <a> <b>

D. Sleep Changes
   Bedtime: __________
   Wakeup: __________
   1. <a> <b> <c>
   2. <a> <b>

E. Psychomotor Changes
   1. <a> <b> <c> <d>
   2. <a> <b>

F. Low Energy
   1. <a> <b> <c> <d>

G. Guilt
   1. <a> <b> <c> <d>
   2. <a> <b>

H. Impaired Concentration
   1. <a> <b> <c> <d> <e>
   2. < >

I. Hopelessness
   1. <a> <b> <c>

J. Morbid/Suicidal Thoughts
   1. <a> <b>
   2. <a> <b> <c> <d> <e>

____
____
____
____
____

DEP/DYS (MDD/DD)

Criteria

If A &/or B & ≥5 of A–H or J,
then criteria met
MDD < >

If A & ≥2 of C, D, F, G, H, or I,
then criteria met
DD < >

Duration

1. ______________ (years old)
2. < > ____________ (years old)
3. MDD < > ________ (weeks)
   DD < > ________ (months)

*DUR met for MDD < >
*DUR met for DD < >

Impairment

1. < > home
2. < > school
3. < > peers

MAN/HYPOMAN

A. Elevated Mood
   1. <a> ______________________
      <b> ______________________
      <c> ______________________
   2. < > ______________________

B. Other Symptoms
   1. <a> ______________________
      <b>
   2. <a> <b> <c> ____________
   3. <a> <b> <c> <d>
   4. <a> <b> <c>
   5. < >
   6. <a> <b> <c> <d> <e>
   7. <a> <b> <c> <d>

C. Interference
   1. < >
   2. < >

Criteria

If A1(a, b, & c) + ≥3 in B + ≥1 in C
or
A2 + ≥4 in B + ≥1 in C,
then criteria met
MAN < >

If A1(a, b, & c) + ≥3 in B +
none in C
or
A2 + ≥4 in B + none in C,
then criteria met
HYPOMAN < >

Duration

1. ______________ (years old)
2. < > ____________ (years old)
3. MAN < > ________ (weeks)
   HYPO < > ________ (days)

*DUR met for MAN < >
*DUR met for HYPOMAN < >

Impairment

1. < > home
2. < > school
3. < > peers

ENU

1. < >
2. <a> <b>
3. <a> <b>

Criteria

If 1, ≥1 in 2, 3a, and 3b, then criteria met
ENU < >

Duration

1. ____________ (years old)
2. < > _________ (years old)
3. <a> _________ (x/week)
   <b> _________ (months)

*DUR met for ENU < >

Impairment

1. < > home
2. < > school
3. < > peers

Type

Nocturnal < >
Diurnal < >
Both < >

ENC

1. < >
2. < >

Criteria

If both 1 & 2, then criteria met
ENC < >

Duration

1. ____________ (years old)
2. < > _________ (years old)
3. <a> _________ (x/month)
   <b> _________ (months)

*DUR met for ENC < >

Impairment

1. < > home
2. < > school
3. < > peers

SCZ/PSY

A. Psychotic Symptoms
1. <a> <b> <c> <d> <e>
2. <a> <b> <c> <d> <e> <f>
3. < >
4. < >
5. < >

B. Interference
1. < >
2. < >
3. < >

Criteria

If ≥2 in A and ≥1 in B, then criteria met
SCZ < >

If ≥1 in A, then criteria met
PSY < >

Duration

1. ______________ (years old)
2. < > ___________ (years old)
3. < > ___________ (months)

*DUR met for SCZ < >
*DUR met for PSY < >

Impairment

1. < > home
2. < > school
3. < > peers

STRESSORS

A. Child Abuse/Neglect
1. <a> <b> <c>
2. <a> <b> <c> <d>
3. <a> <b> <c> <d>
4. < >
5. < >

Duration

1. ______________________
2. < > ___________________
3. ______________________
4. ______________________
5. < >

B. Other Stressors
1. <a> <b> <c> <d> <e>
2. < >
3. <a> <b>
4. <a> <b> <c>
5. <a> <b>
6. <a> <b>
7. <a> __________________
   <b>
8. <a> <b> <c> <d>
9. < > __________________
   ____
   ____
10. < >
11. < > _________________
   ____
   ____

P-ChIPS Scoring Form
Profile Sheet

Child's Number: ______________________ Date: ______________

Child's Name: ______________________ Time Started: ______________

Date of Birth: ______________ Age: ______________ Time Ended: ______________

Race: ______________ Sex: ______________ Interviewer: ______________

Informant's Name: ______________________

Informant's Relationship (circle one): Mother, Father, Stepmother, Stepfather, Guardian, Other: ______________

	Disorder	Symptoms	Diagnosis	Duration	Clinician's Diagnosis
ADHD	**Attention-Deficit/Hyperactivity Disorder**	<>	<>	<>	**Axis I**
	Type: Inattentive, Hyperactive–Impulsive, Combined				
ODD	**Oppositional Defiant Disorder**	<>	<>	<>	
CD	**Conduct Disorder**	<>	<>	<>	
	Onset: Childhood, Adolescent				
	Severity: Mild, Moderate, Severe				
SUBAB	**Substance Abuse**	<>	<>	<>	
	Substance(s): ______________				
PHO	**Specific Phobia**	<>	<>	<>	**Axis II**
	Type: ______________				
SOCPHO	**Social Phobia**	<>	<>	<>	
SEPANX	**Separation Anxiety Disorder**	<>	<>	<>	**Axis III**
GENANX	**General Anxiety Disorder**	<>	<>	<>	
OCD	**Obsessive-Compulsive Disorder**	<>	<>	<>	
PTSD	**Posttraumatic Stress Disorder**	<>	<>	<>	**Axis IV**
	Type: Acute, Chronic				
	Onset: Regular, Delayed				
ASD	**Acute Stress Disorder**	<>	<>	<>	
ANO	**Anorexia**	<>	<>	<>	**Axis V**
BUL	**Bulimia**	<>	<>	<>	**current:**
DEP	**Major Depressive Disorder**	<>	<>	<>	**past year:**
DYS	**Dysthymic Disorder**	<>	<>	<>	
MAN	**Mania**	<>	<>	<>	
HYPOMAN	**Hypomania**	<>	<>	<>	
ENU	**Enuresis**	<>	<>	<>	
	Type: Nocturnal, Diurnal, Both				
ENC	**Encopresis**	<>	<>	<>	
SCZ	**Schizophrenia**	<>	<>	<>	
PSY	**Psychosis**	<>	<>	<>	

Psychosocial Stressors:

Other Stressors:

Behavioral Observations

Appearance:

Affect:

Effort:

Level of Activity:

Unusual Behaviors:

Presenting Problem

Home

1.

2.

School

1.

2.

3.

4.

5.

Peers/Work

1.

2.

3.

4.

5.

Medication

Type:

Dosage:

Child's Name: ______________________________

Date: ________________

ADHD	ODD	CD
A. Inattention 1. <a> <b> 2. < > 3. <a> <b> 4. <a> <b> <c> 5. < > 6. < > 7. < > 8. <a> <b> 9. <a> <b> B. Hyperactivity–Impulsivity 1. <a> <b> 2. <a> <b> 3. < > 4. <a> <b> 5. < > 6. <a> <b> 7. < > 8. <a> <b> 9. <a> <b> <c>	1. <a> <b> 2. <a> <b> 3. <a> <b> <c> <d> 4. < > 5. <a> <b> 6. < > 7. < > 8. < >	1. < > 2. <a> <b> 3. < > 4. < > 5. < > 6. < > 7. <a> <b> 8. <a> <b> 9. < > 10. <a> <b> 11. < > 12. < > 13. < > 14. < > 15. <a> <b>
Criteria If ≥6 in *A only*, then criteria met Inattentive < > If ≥6 in *B only*, then criteria met Hyperactive–Impulsive < > If ≥6 in A *and* ≥6 in B, then criteria met Combined < >	**Criteria** If ≥4, then criteria met ODD < >	**Criteria** If ≥3, then criteria met CD < >
Duration 1. ____________ (years old) 2. < > _________ (years old) 3. < > __________ (months) * DUR met for ADHD < >	**Duration** 1. ____________ (years old) 2. < > _________ (years old) 3. < > __________ (months) * DUR met for ODD < >	**Duration** 1. ____________ (years old) 2. < > _________ (years old) 3. < > __________ (months) * DUR met for CD < >
Impairment 1. < > home 2. < > school 3. < > peers	**Impairment** 1. < > home 2. < > school 3. < > peers	**Impairment** 1. < > home 2. < > school 3. < > peers **Type** Childhood Onset < > Adolescent Onset < > Mild < > Moderate < > Severe < >

SUB AB	PHO	SOCIAL PHO
1. < > <a>____________ <b>____________ <c>____________ ____________ 2. < > ____________ 3. < > ____________ 4. < > ____________	1. ____________ ____________ ____________ 2. <a> <b> 3. <a> <b> 4. <ai> <aii> <aiii> <aiv> <b> 5. <a> <b>	1. <a> <b> 2. < > 3. <a> <b> 4. <ai> <aii> <aiii> <aiv> <b> 5. < >
Duration 1. ________ (years old) 2. < > ________ (years old) ________ (months) * DUR met for SUB AB < >	**Criteria** If 1–4, then criteria met PHO < >	**Criteria** If 1–4, then criteria met SOCIAL PHO < >
	Duration 1. ________ (years old) 2. < > ________ (years old) 3. < > ________ (months) * DUR met for PHO < >	**Duration** 1. ________ (years old) 2. < > ________ (years old) 3. < > ________ (months) *DUR met for SOCIAL PHO < >
Impairment 1. <a> <b> 2. < > 3. <a> <b> 4. < >	**Impairment** 1. < > home 2. < > school 3. < > peers	**Impairment** 1. < > home 2. < > school 3. < > peers
Criteria If any use (Q1–4) and any impairment (1–4), then criteria met SUB AB < >	**Type(s)** Animal < > Natural Environment < > Blood–Injection–Injury < > Situational < > Other ____________ < >	
Type(s) ____________ ____________ ____________ ____________		

SEP ANX	GEN ANX	OCD
1. <a> <b> 2. <a> <b> 3. < > 4. <a> <b> 5. <a> <b> 6. <a> <b> 7. <a> <b> 8. <a> <b>	1. < > ____________ ____________ ____________ ____________ ____________ 2. <a> <b> 3. <a> <b> <c> <d> <e> <f>	A. Compulsions 1. < > ____________ 2. <a> ____________ <b> 3. < > B. Obsessions 1. <a> ____________ <b> ____________ <c> ____________ 2. <a> <b> <c> 3. < > C. Interference 1. <a> <b> <c>
Criteria If ≥3, then criteria met SEP ANX < >	**Criteria** If 1–3, then criteria met GEN ANX < >	**Criteria** If A1, A2, & C, then criteria met Compulsions < > If B1, B2, & C, then criteria met Obsessions < > If Compulsions + and/or Obsessions +, then criteria met OCD < >
Duration 1. ____________ (years old) 2. < > ____________ (years old) 3. < > ____________ (weeks) *DUR met for SEP ANX < >	**Duration** 1. ____________ (years old) 2. < > ____________ (years old) 3. < > ____________ (months) *DUR met for GEN ANX < >	**Duration** 1. ____________ (years old) 2. < > ____________ (years old) ____________ (months) *DUR met for OCD < >
Impairment 1. < > home 2. < > school 3. < > peers	**Impairment** 1. < > home 2. < > school 3. < > peers	**Impairment** 1. < > home 2. < > school 3. < > peers

STRESS (ASD/PTSD)	ANO	BUL
A. Exposure 1. <a> <b> ______________ 2. <a> <b> <c> <d> <e> 3. < > ______________ B. Dissociation 1. <a> <b> <c> <d> 2. < > 3. < > 4. < > 5. < > C. Reexperiencing 1. <a> <b> <c> 2. <a> <b> 3. <a> <b> 4. <a> <b> 5. < > D. Avoidance 1. <a> <b> 2. <a> <b> <c> 3. < > 4. <a> <b> 5. <a> <b> 6. <a> <b> 7. <a> <b> E. Hyperarousal 1. <a> <b> 2. <a> <b> 3. < > 4. < > 5. < >	1. <a> <b> 2. <a> ht: __________ wt: __________ <b> ht: __________ wt: __________ 3. <a> <b> <c> 4. <a> <b> <c> 5. < >	1. < > ______________ ______________ 2. <a> <b> <c> <d> 3. <a> <b> <c> <d> 4. <a> <b>
Criteria If A1 & A2, ≥3 in B, ≥1 in C, ≥3 in D, and ≥2 in E, then criteria met ASD < > If A1 & A2, ≥1 in C, ≥3 in D, and ≥2 in E, then criteria met PTSD < >	**Criteria** If 1–4 (&5 for pubescent girls), then criteria met ANO < >	**Criteria** If 1–4, then criteria met BUL < >
Duration 1. __________ (years old) 2. < > ________ (years old) 3. a. < > ______ (weeks) b. < > c. < > ______ (days) 4. < > ________ (months) *DUR met for ASD < > *DUR met for PTSD < >	**Duration** 1. ________ (years old) 2. < > ______ (years old) 3. < > ______ (months) *DUR met for ANO < >	**Duration** 1. ________ (years old) 2. < > ______ (years old) 3. a. < > ____ (#/week) b. < > ____ (months) *DUR met for BUL < >
Impairment 1. < > home 2. < > school 3. < > peers **Type (PTSD)** Acute < > Regular Onset < > Chronic < > Delayed Onset < >	**Impairment** 1. < > home 2. < > school 3. < > peers	**Impairment** 1. < > home 2. < > school 3. < > peers

DEP/DYS (MDD/DD)

A. Dysphoric Mood
1. <a> <b> <c>
2. <a> <bi> <bii> <biii> <c> <d>

B. Loss of Interest
1. <a> <b>
2. <a> <b> <c>

C. Appetite Changes
1. <a> <b> <c>
2. <a> <b>

D. Sleep Changes
Bedtime: __________
Wakeup: __________
1. <a> <b> <c>
2. <a> <b>

E. Psychomotor Changes
1. <a> <b> <c> <d>
2. <a> <b>

F. Low Energy
1. <a> <b> <c> <d>

G. Guilt
1. <a> <b> <c> <d>
2. <a> <b>

H. Impaired Concentration
1. <a> <b> <c> <d> <e>
2. < >

I. Hopelessness
1. <a> <b> <c>

J. Morbid/Suicidal Thoughts
1. <a> <b>
2. <a> <b> <c> <d> <e>

____
____
____
____
____

DEP/DYS (MDD/DD)

Criteria
If A &/or B & ≥5 of A–H or J,
then criteria met
MDD < >

If A & ≥2 of C, D, F, G, H, or I,
then criteria met
DD < >

Duration
1. ______________ (years old)
2. < > ______________ (years old)
3. MDD < > ________ (weeks)
DD < > ________ (months)

*DUR met for MDD < >
*DUR met for DD < >

Impairment
1. < > home
2. < > school
3. < > peers

MAN/HYPOMAN

A. Elevated Mood
1. <a> ______________________
<b> ______________________
<c> ______________________
2. < > ______________________

B. Other Symptoms
1. <a> ______________________
<b>
2. <a> <b> <c> ____________
3. <a> <b> <c> <d>
4. <a> <b> <c>
5. < >
6. <a> <b> <c> <d> <e>
7. <a> <b> <c> <d>

C. Interference
1. < >
2. < >

Criteria
If A1(a, b, & c) + ≥3 in B + ≥1 in C
or
A2 + ≥4 in B + ≥1 in C,
then criteria met
MAN < >

If A1(a, b, & c) + ≥3 in B +
none in C
or
A2 + ≥4 in B + none in C,
then criteria met
HYPOMAN < >

Duration
1. ______________ (years old)
2. < > ______________ (years old)
3. MAN < > ________ (weeks)
HYPO < > ________ (days)

*DUR met for MAN < >
*DUR met for HYPOMAN < >

Impairment
1. < > home
2. < > school
3. < > peers

ENU

1. < >
2. <a> <b>
3. <a> <b>

Criteria
If 1, ≥1 in 2, 3a, and 3b, then criteria met
ENU < >

Duration
1. ____________ (years old)
2. < > _________ (years old)
3. <a> _________ (x/week)
   <b> _________ (months)

*DUR met for ENU < >

Impairment
1. < > home
2. < > school
3. < > peers

Type

Nocturnal	< >
Diurnal	< >
Both	< >

ENC

1. < >
2. < >

Criteria
If both 1 & 2, then criteria met
ENC < >

Duration
1. ____________ (years old)
2. < > _________ (years old)
3. <a> _________ (x/month)
   <b> _________ (months)

*DUR met for ENC < >

Impairment
1. < > home
2. < > school
3. < > peers

SCZ/PSY

A. Psychotic Symptoms
1. <a> <b> <c> <d> <e>
2. <a> <b> <c> <d> <e> <f>
3. < >
4. < >
5. < >

B. Interference
1. < >
2. < >
3. < >

Criteria
If ≥2 in A and ≥1 in B, then criteria met
SCZ < >

If ≥1 in A, then criteria met
PSY < >

Duration
1. ____________ (years old)
2. < > _________ (years old)
3. < > _________ (months)

*DUR met for SCZ < >
*DUR met for PSY < >

Impairment
1. < > home
2. < > school
3. < > peers

STRESSORS

A. Child Abuse/Neglect
1. <a> <b> <c>
2. <a> <b> <c> <d>
3. <a> <b> <c> <d>
4. < >
5. < >

Duration
1. ____________
2. < > ____________
3. ____________
4. ____________
5. < >

B. Other Stressors
1. <a> <b> <c> <d> <e>
2. < >
3. <a> <b>
4. <a> <b> <c>
5. <a> <b>
6. <a> <b>
7. <a> ____________
   <b>
8. <a> <b> <c> <d>
9. < > ____________
10. < >
11. < > ____________

P-ChIPS Scoring Form
Profile Sheet

Child's Number: ______________________________ Date: ______________

Child's Name: ______________________________ Time Started: ______________

Date of Birth: ______________ Age: ______________ Time Ended: ______________

Race: ______________ Sex: ______________ Interviewer: ______________

Informant's Name: ______________________________

Informant's Relationship (circle one): Mother, Father, Stepmother, Stepfather, Guardian, Other: ______________

	Disorder	Symptoms	Diagnosis	Duration	Clinician's Diagnosis
ADHD	**Attention-Deficit/Hyperactivity Disorder** *Type:* Inattentive, Hyperactive–Impulsive, Combined	<>	<>	<>	**Axis I**
ODD	**Oppositional Defiant Disorder**	<>	<>	<>	
CD	**Conduct Disorder** *Onset:* Childhood, Adolescent *Severity:* Mild, Moderate, Severe	<>	<>	<>	
SUBAB	**Substance Abuse** *Substance(s):* ______________	<>	<>	<>	
PHO	**Specific Phobia** *Type:* ______________	<>	<>	<>	**Axis II**
SOCPHO	**Social Phobia**	<>	<>	<>	
SEPANX	**Separation Anxiety Disorder**	<>	<>	<>	**Axis III**
GENANX	**General Anxiety Disorder**	<>	<>	<>	
OCD	**Obsessive-Compulsive Disorder**	<>	<>	<>	
PTSD	**Posttraumatic Stress Disorder** *Type:* Acute, Chronic *Onset:* Regular, Delayed	<>	<>	<>	**Axis IV**
ASD	**Acute Stress Disorder**	<>	<>	<>	
ANO	**Anorexia**	<>	<>	<>	**Axis V**
BUL	**Bulimia**	<>	<>	<>	**current:**
DEP	**Major Depressive Disorder**	<>	<>	<>	**past year:**
DYS	**Dysthymic Disorder**	<>	<>	<>	
MAN	**Mania**	<>	<>	<>	
HYPOMAN	**Hypomania**	<>	<>	<>	
ENU	**Enuresis** *Type:* Nocturnal, Diurnal, Both	<>	<>	<>	
ENC	**Encopresis**	<>	<>	<>	
SCZ	**Schizophrenia**	<>	<>	<>	
PSY	**Psychosis**	<>	<>	<>	

Psychosocial Stressors:

Other Stressors:

Behavioral Observations

Appearance:

Affect:

Effort:

Level of Activity:

Unusual Behaviors:

Presenting Problem

Home

1.

2.

School

1.

2.

3.

4.

5.

Peers/Work

1.

2.

3.

4.

5.

Medication

Type:

Dosage:

Child's Name: ______________________________

Date: ________________

ADHD	ODD	CD
A. Inattention 1. <a> <b> 2. < > 3. <a> <b> 4. <a> <b> <c> 5. < > 6. < > 7. < > 8. <a> <b> 9. <a> <b> B. Hyperactivity–Impulsivity 1. <a> <b> 2. <a> <b> 3. < > 4. <a> <b> 5. < > 6. <a> <b> 7. < > 8. <a> <b> 9. <a> <b> <c>	1. <a> <b> 2. <a> <b> 3. <a> <b> <c> <d> 4. < > 5. <a> <b> 6. < > 7. < > 8. < >	1. < > 2. <a> <b> 3. < > 4. < > 5. < > 6. < > 7. <a> <b> 8. <a> <b> 9. < > 10. <a> <b> 11. < > 12. < > 13. < > 14. < > 15. <a> <b>
Criteria If ≥6 in *A only*, then criteria met Inattentive < > If ≥6 in *B only*, then criteria met Hyperactive–Impulsive < > If ≥6 in A *and* ≥6 in B, then criteria met Combined < >	**Criteria** If ≥4, then criteria met ODD < >	**Criteria** If ≥3, then criteria met CD < >
Duration 1. ____________ (years old) 2. < > _________ (years old) 3. < > __________ (months) * DUR met for ADHD < >	**Duration** 1. ____________ (years old) 2. < > _________ (years old) 3. < > __________ (months) * DUR met for ODD < >	**Duration** 1. ____________ (years old) 2. < > _________ (years old) 3. < > __________ (months) * DUR met for CD < >
Impairment 1. < > home 2. < > school 3. < > peers	**Impairment** 1. < > home 2. < > school 3. < > peers	**Impairment** 1. < > home 2. < > school 3. < > peers
		Type Childhood Onset < > Adolescent Onset < > Mild < > Moderate < > Severe < >

SUB AB

1. < >
   <a>____________________
   <b>____________________
   <c>____________________
   ____
2. < > ____________________
3. < > ____________________
4. < > ____________________

Duration

1. ____________ (years old)
2. < > __________ (years old)
   __________ (months)

* DUR met for SUB AB < >

Impairment

1. <a> <b>
2. < >
3. <a> <b>
4. < >

Criteria

If any use (Q1–4) and any impairment (1–4), then criteria met SUB AB < >

Type(s) ____________________
____
____
____

PHO

1. ____________________
   ____
   ____
2. <a> <b>
3. <a> <b>
4. <ai> <aii> <aiii> <aiv> <b>
5. <a> <b>

Criteria

If 1–4, then criteria met
PHO < >

Duration

1. ____________ (years old)
2. < > __________ (years old)
3. < > __________ (months)

* DUR met for PHO < >

Impairment

1. < > home
2. < > school
3. < > peers

Type(s)

Animal	< >
Natural Environment	< >
Blood–Injection–Injury	< >
Situational	< >
Other ________________	< >

SOCIAL PHO

1. <a> <b>
2. < >
3. <a> <b>
4. <ai> <aii> <aiii> <aiv> <b>
5. < >

Criteria

If 1–4, then criteria met
SOCIAL PHO < >

Duration

1. ____________ (years old)
2. < > __________ (years old)
3. < > __________ (months)

*DUR met for SOCIAL PHO < >

Impairment

1. < > home
2. < > school
3. < > peers

SEP ANX	GEN ANX	OCD
1. <a> <b> 2. <a> <b> 3. < > 4. <a> <b> 5. <a> <b> 6. <a> <b> 7. <a> <b> 8. <a> <b>	1. < > ______________ ______________ ______________ ______________ ______________ 2. <a> <b> 3. <a> <b> <c> <d> <e> <f>	A. Compulsions 1. < > ____________ 2. <a> ____________ <b> 3. < > B. Obsessions 1. <a> ____________ <b> ____________ <c> ____________ 2. <a> <b> <c> 3. < > C. Interference 1. <a> <b> <c>
Criteria If ≥3, then criteria met SEP ANX < >	**Criteria** If 1–3, then criteria met GEN ANX < >	**Criteria** If A1, A2, & C, then criteria met Compulsions < > If B1, B2, & C, then criteria met Obsessions < > If Compulsions + and/or Obsessions +, then criteria met OCD < >
Duration 1. ____________ (years old) 2. < > __________ (years old) 3. < > __________ (weeks) *DUR met for SEP ANX < >	**Duration** 1. ____________ (years old) 2. < > __________ (years old) 3. < > __________ (months) *DUR met for GEN ANX < >	**Duration** 1. ____________ (years old) 2. < > __________ (years old) __________ (months) *DUR met for OCD < >
Impairment 1. < > home 2. < > school 3. < > peers	**Impairment** 1. < > home 2. < > school 3. < > peers	**Impairment** 1. < > home 2. < > school 3. < > peers

STRESS (ASD/PTSD)	ANO	BUL
A. Exposure 1. <a> <b> ______ 2. <a> <b> <c> <d> <e> 3. < > ______ B. Dissociation 1. <a> <b> <c> <d> 2. < > 3. < > 4. < > 5. < > C. Reexperiencing 1. <a> <b> <c> 2. <a> <b> 3. <a> <b> 4. <a> <b> 5. < > D. Avoidance 1. <a> <b> 2. <a> <b> <c> 3. < > 4. <a> <b> 5. <a> <b> 6. <a> <b> 7. <a> <b> E. Hyperarousal 1. <a> <b> 2. <a> <b> 3. < > 4. < > 5. < >	1. <a> <b> 2. <a> ht: ______ wt: ______ <b> ht: ______ wt: ______ 3. <a> <b> <c> 4. <a> <b> <c> 5. < >	1. < > ______ ______ 2. <a> <b> <c> <d> 3. <a> <b> <c> <d> 4. <a> <b>
Criteria If A1 & A2, ≥3 in B, ≥1 in C, ≥3 in D, and ≥2 in E, then criteria met ASD < > If A1 & A2, ≥1 in C, ≥3 in D, and ≥2 in E, then criteria met PTSD < >	**Criteria** If 1–4 (&5 for pubescent girls), then criteria met ANO < >	**Criteria** If 1–4, then criteria met BUL < >
Duration 1. ______ (years old) 2. < > ______ (years old) 3. a. < > ______ (weeks) b. < > c. < > ______ (days) 4. < > ______ (months) *DUR met for ASD < > *DUR met for PTSD < >	**Duration** 1. ______ (years old) 2. < > ______ (years old) 3. < > ______ (months) *DUR met for ANO < >	**Duration** 1. ______ (years old) 2. < > ______ (years old) 3. a. < > ______ (#/week) b. < > ______ (months) *DUR met for BUL < >
Impairment 1. < > home 2. < > school 3. < > peers **Type (PTSD)** Acute < > Regular Onset < > Chronic < > Delayed Onset < >	**Impairment** 1. < > home 2. < > school 3. < > peers	**Impairment** 1. < > home 2. < > school 3. < > peers

DEP/DYS (MDD/DD)

A. Dysphoric Mood
1. <a> <b> <c>
2. <a> <bi> <bii> <biii> <c> <d>

B. Loss of Interest
1. <a> <b>
2. <a> <b> <c>

C. Appetite Changes
1. <a> <b> <c>
2. <a> <b>

D. Sleep Changes
Bedtime: ____________
Wakeup: ____________
1. <a> <b> <c>
2. <a> <b>

E. Psychomotor Changes
1. <a> <b> <c> <d>
2. <a> <b>

F. Low Energy
1. <a> <b> <c> <d>

G. Guilt
1. <a> <b> <c> <d>
2. <a> <b>

H. Impaired Concentration
1. <a> <b> <c> <d> <e>
2. < >

I. Hopelessness
1. <a> <b> <c>

J. Morbid/Suicidal Thoughts
1. <a> <b>
2. <a> <b> <c> <d> <e>

____
____
____
____
____

DEP/DYS (MDD/DD)

Criteria

If A &/or B & ≥5 of A–H or J,
then criteria met
MDD < >

If A & ≥2 of C, D, F, G, H, or I,
then criteria met
DD < >

Duration

1. ______________ (years old)
2. < > ____________ (years old)
3. MDD < > ________ (weeks)
   DD < > ________ (months)

*DUR met for MDD < >
*DUR met for DD < >

Impairment

1. < > home
2. < > school
3. < > peers

MAN/HYPOMAN

A. Elevated Mood
1. <a> ____________________
   <b> ____________________
   <c> ____________________
2. < > ____________________

B. Other Symptoms
1. <a> ____________________
   <b>
2. <a> <b> <c> ____________
3. <a> <b> <c> <d>
4. <a> <b> <c>
5. < >
6. <a> <b> <c> <d> <e>
7. <a> <b> <c> <d>

C. Interference
1. < >
2. < >

Criteria

If A1(a, b, & c) + ≥3 in B + ≥1 in C
or
A2 + ≥4 in B + ≥1 in C,
then criteria met
MAN < >

If A1(a, b, & c) + ≥3 in B +
none in C
or
A2 + ≥4 in B + none in C,
then criteria met
HYPOMAN < >

Duration

1. ______________ (years old)
2. < > ____________ (years old)
3. MAN < > ________ (weeks)
   HYPO < > ________ (days)

*DUR met for MAN < >
*DUR met for HYPOMAN < >

Impairment

1. < > home
2. < > school
3. < > peers

ENU

1. < >
2. <a> <b>
3. <a> <b>

Criteria

If 1, ≥1 in 2, 3a, and 3b,
then criteria met
ENU < >

Duration

1. ____________ (years old)
2. < > __________ (years old)
3. <a> __________ (x/week)
   <b> __________ (months)

*DUR met for ENU < >

Impairment

1. < > home
2. < > school
3. < > peers

Type

Nocturnal < >
Diurnal < >
Both < >

ENC

1. < >
2. < >

Criteria

If both 1 & 2, then criteria met
ENC < >

Duration

1. ____________ (years old)
2. < > __________ (years old)
3. <a> __________ (x/month)
   <b> __________ (months)

*DUR met for ENC < >

Impairment

1. < > home
2. < > school
3. < > peers

SCZ/PSY

A. Psychotic Symptoms
1. <a> <b> <c> <d> <e>
2. <a> <b> <c> <d> <e> <f>
3. < >
4. < >
5. < >

B. Interference
1. < >
2. < >
3. < >

Criteria

If ≥2 in A and ≥1 in B,
then criteria met
SCZ < >

If ≥1 in A, then criteria met
PSY < >

Duration

1. ____________ (years old)
2. < > __________ (years old)
3. < > __________ (months)

*DUR met for SCZ < >
*DUR met for PSY < >

Impairment

1. < > home
2. < > school
3. < > peers

STRESSORS

A. Child Abuse/Neglect
1. <a> <b> <c>
2. <a> <b> <c> <d>
3. <a> <b> <c> <d>
4. < >
5. < >

Duration

1. ____________
2. < > ____________
3. ____________
4. ____________
5. < >

B. Other Stressors
1. <a> <b> <c> <d> <e>
2. < >
3. <a> <b>
4. <a> <b> <c>
5. <a> <b>
6. <a> <b>
7. <a> ____________
   <b>
8. <a> <b> <c> <d>
9. < > ____________
   ____
   ____
10. < >
11. < > ____________
   ____
   ____